Contents

Preface v

Section A - Common transient neonatal disorders

1. Birth injuries 1

2. Skin/mucous membrane disorders 9

3. Miscellaneous 19

Section B - System abnormalities

4. Skin 23

5. Head and neck 47

6. Neurology 75

7. Cardiothoracic 87

8. Gastrointestinal and genito-urinary 97

9. Skeletal 117

10. Syndromes 139

11. Endocrine 147

12. Problems particular to the premature infant 151

13. Neonatal tumours 165

14. Iatrogenic 173

Index 181

Acknowledgements

We would like to express our gratitude for the generosity of our colleagues in contributing photographs we were lacking.

Special thanks to the following who have made significant contributions within their fields of expertise:

Dr N Bridges
Dr R Chinn
Miss PC Lin
Dr M Phelan
Mr N Waterhouse, Mr B Coughlan & Mr R Carr

Thanks to the photographic department of Chelsea and Westminster Hospital without whom this project would not have succeeded.

We would also like to thank the staff of the Neonatal Unit at Chelsea and Westminster Hospital for their assistance and patience.

Special thanks to Gina Almond and Jane Tozer of Mosby for all their expert help and for keeping us under control.

Finally we are indebted to all the parents for allowing us to photograph their infants.

List of Contributors

Dr A Bedford-Russell, Dept of Child Health, St George's Hospital Medical School, London
3.6, 4.4c, 4.21c, 5.13a, 5.18, 5.22a–b, 5.31, 5.32a–b, 6.5, 8.1, 9.8,

Dr N Bridges, Dept of Paediatrics, Chelsea & Westminster Hospital, London
11.2c

Dr M Brueton, Dept of Paediatrics, Chelsea & Westminster Hospital, London
13.6b

Dr R Chinn, Dept of Radiology, Chelsea & Westminster Hospital, London
9.14a, 12.1–12.3, 12.8e–f.

Craniofacial Unit, Chelsea & Westminster Hospital, London
5.1, 5.2b–c, 5.4a–c, 5.5, 5.19, 5.20a–b, 5.23a–b, 5.24a–c, 5.25a, 9.2a, 9.2d, 9.9a, 9.17a–b, 10.8.

Mr M Haddad, Dept of Paediatric Surgery, Chelsea & Westminster Hospital, London
8.2, 8.3, 8.8b, 8.8f, 8.10c, 8.11d.

Dr P Hamilton, Dept of Child Health, St George's Hospital Medical School, London
1.1, 1.5, 1.8a ,3.1, 3.2, 4.14, 4.18a–b, 5.30, 6.8, 6.9a–b, 7.2c, 8.12b, 9.11a-b, 10.1, 10.3b, 13.2a-b

Miss A Hulme, Dept of Orthopaedic Surgery, Chelsea & Westminster Hospital, London
1.8b.

Mr R Knowlden, Dept of Ophthalmology, Chelsea & Westminster Hospital, London
5.9, 5.13b, 5.14–5.16.

Dr I Z Kovar, Dept of Child Health, Chelsea & Westminster Hospital, London
1.6, 3.3, 4.7a–b, 4.19, 4.20, 5.12, 6.1, 7.1, 7.7a, 7.9, 7.10, 9.13c, 9.18, 10.3a, 10.9, 12.5a-b, 13.3.

Dr S Mayou, Dept of Dermatology, Chelsea & Westminster Hospital, London
4.1, 4.2, 4.4b, 4.9, 4.12a–b, 6.6b, 7.3a–b, 8.13, 9.7, 10.6a–b.

Mr I Mustaq, Dept of Surgery, Institute of Child Health, London
8.4

Dr M Phelan, Dept of Radiology, Chelsea & Westminster Hospital, London
9.14a, 12.1–12.3, 12.8e–f.

Dr J Shaw, Dept of Paediatrics, University College Hospital, London
4.1, 4.2, 4.4b, 4.9, 4.12a–b, 6.6b, 7.3a–b, 8.13, 9.7, 10.6a–b.

Neonatology

Mi
BSc,
Con
Chel
Lon

Related titles published in Mosby's Diagnosis in color series:

The Nail in Clinical Diagnosis 2/e: Beaven & Brooks
ENT Diagnosis 3/e: Bull
Infectious Diseases 3/e: Emond, Rowland & Welsby
Surgical Diagnosis: Greig
Medical Microbiology: Hart & Shears
Breast Diseases: Mansel & Bundred
Medical Mycology: Midgley, Clayton & Hay
Skin Signs in Clinical Medicine: Savin, Hunter & Hepburn
Pediatrics: Taylor & Raffles
Cardiology: Timmis & Brecker
Oro-Facial Diseases 2/e: Tyldesley
Oral Medicine 2/e: Tyldesley
Obstetrics and Gynaecology: Symonds & Macpherson
Levene's Dermatology 2/e: White
STD & AIDS 2/e: Wisdom & Hawkins
Physical Signs in General Medicine 2/e: Zatouroff

Development Editor: **Gina Almond**
Project Manager & Layout: **Jane Tozer**
Design: **Greg Smith**
Cover Design: **Paul Phillips**
Production: **Gudrun Hughes**
Index: **Anita Reid**
Publisher: **Jane Ryley**

MOSBY
An imprint of Elsevier Science Limited
M is a registered trademark of Elsevier Science Limited

Published in 1999 by Mosby
Reprinted 2000, 2002

ISBN 0 7234 3011-X

Printed in China by RDC Group Limited
B/03

Preface

Pattern recognition is a crucial aspect of clinical management, particularly exemplified in relation to neonatal care. Health professionals who work with newborn infants, including paediatricians, midwives, GPs and health visitors, are often faced with clinical appearances unfamiliar to them. This may simply involve a skin rash at one end of the spectrum or multi-system disease e.g. histiocytosis, at the other.

This book brings together all common patterns of presenting illnesses in the newborn, including those which occur transiently, disorders relating to specific systems and finally problems peculiar to the preterm infant. In addition innovative chapters on iatrogenic complications of newborn care and neonatal oncology are included.

We hope that this book will prove a useful addition to book shelves in neonatal units, delivery suites, post-natal wards and emergency departments. It will also be of value within primary care and office-based paediatrics. Both undergraduate and postgraduate students should also find the book an accessible visual guide to common neonatal conditions in preparation for paediatric examinations.

Michael Markiewicz
Ed Abrahamson

To my parents who have loved and supported me throughout my life, and to Terry and my children for all their love and inspiration and for putting up with all the late nights. Finally to our little daughter Leah who never had the chance to enjoy life.

MM

For the unending love and support of my parents and family.

EA

1 Birth injuries

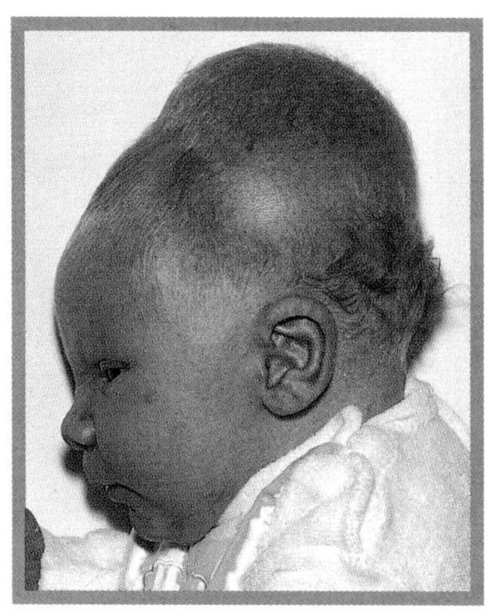

1.1 Cephalohaematoma

These localized scalp swellings are caused by an accumulation of blood between the periosteum and the skull bone and are particularly common after ventouse extraction. If they are extensive, as in the infant shown, they may result in anaemia and neonatal jaundice. Palpation of the margin of the swelling often suggests an underlying depressed fracture but this is only rarely present and a skull radiograph is unnecessary. No treatment is required and resolution usually occurs within 6 weeks. However, it may persist, leaving a hard, calcified swelling.

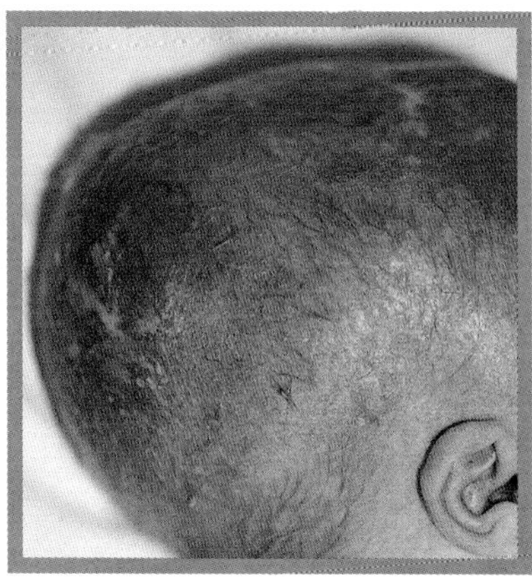

1.2 Caput succedaneum

Caput succedaneum is a diffuse scalp swelling, occasionally associated with discoloration, caused by oedema of the soft tissues of the scalp. Unlike cephalohaematoma, the swelling may cross the mid-line. Caput may also be associated with early jaundice from resorption of extravasated blood.

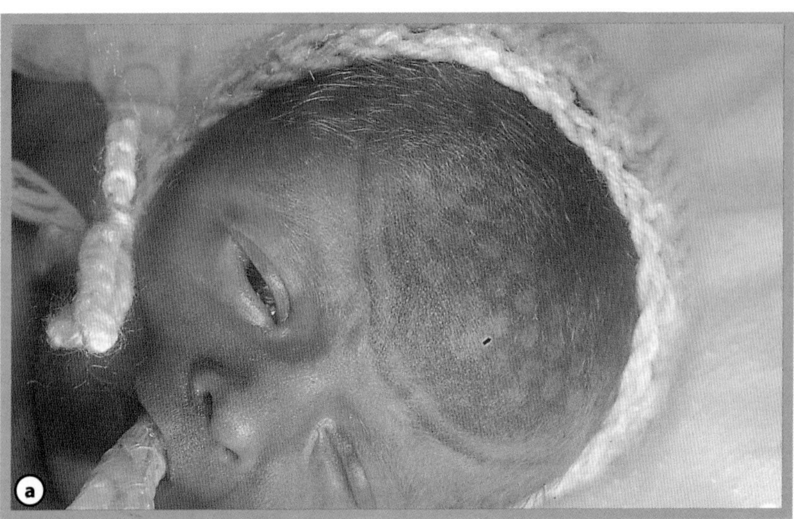

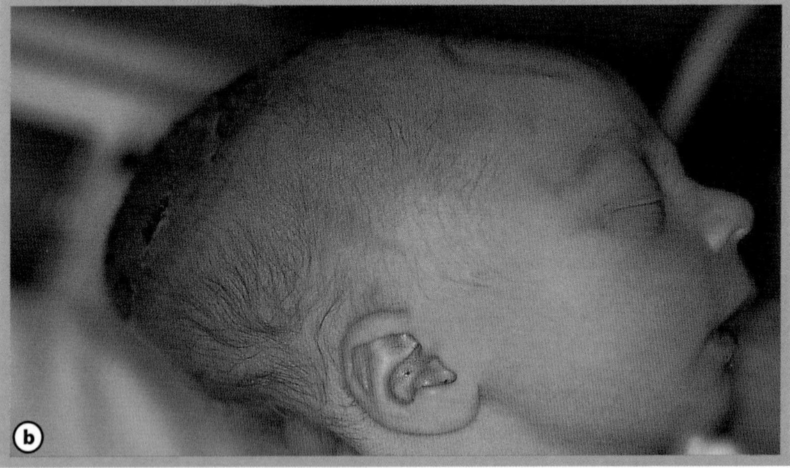

1.3a and 1.3b Ventouse

The ventouse extractor has left telltale marks on the skin which resolved completely after 2 weeks. The second infant's (**1.3b**) head has been clearly misshapen by the effect of suction.

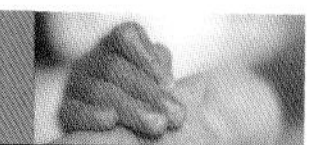

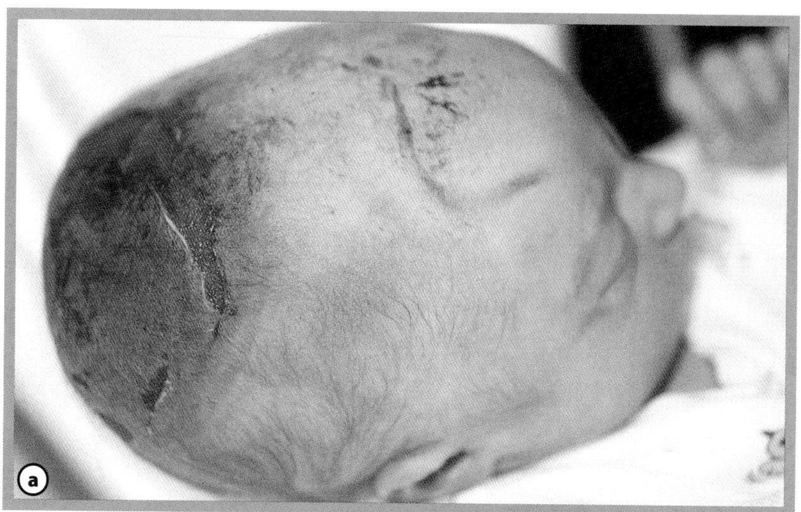

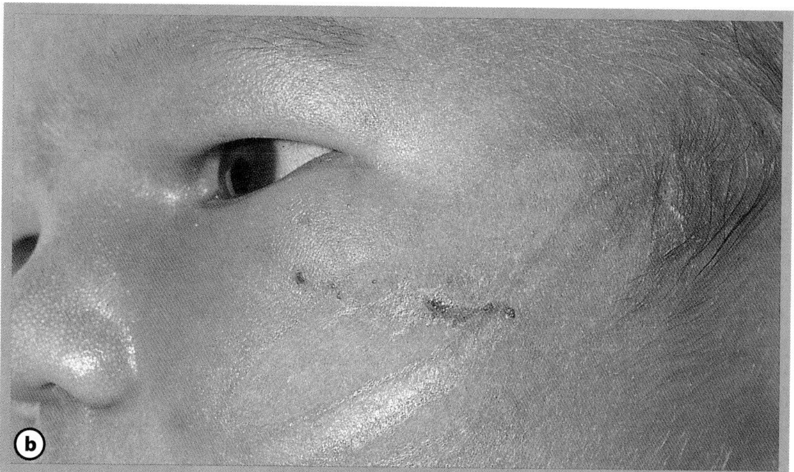

1.4a and 1.4b Forceps marks
The first infant (1.4a) had forceps applied after a failed ventouse. A close-up view of another infant (1.4b) reveals indentation and laceration of the face. However, permanent scarring is very rare from these injuries.

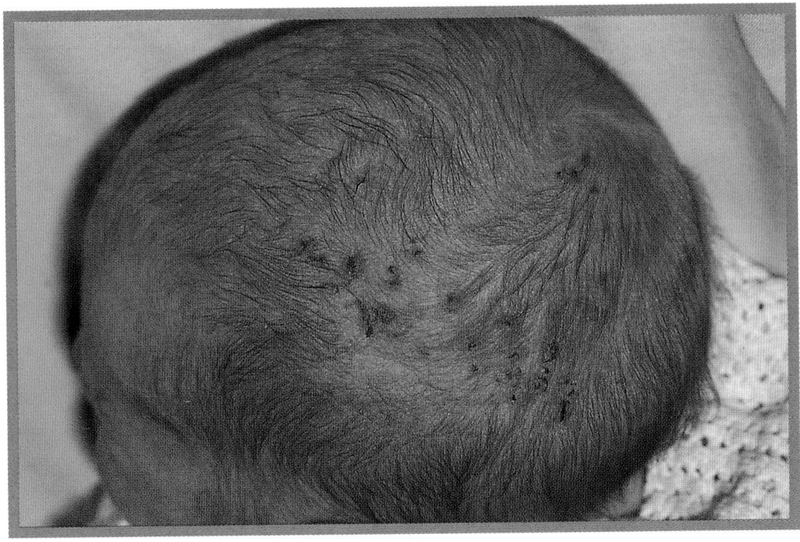

1.5 Foetal scalp electrode burn
Note the scalp lacerations caused by numerous attempts to place a foetal electrode.

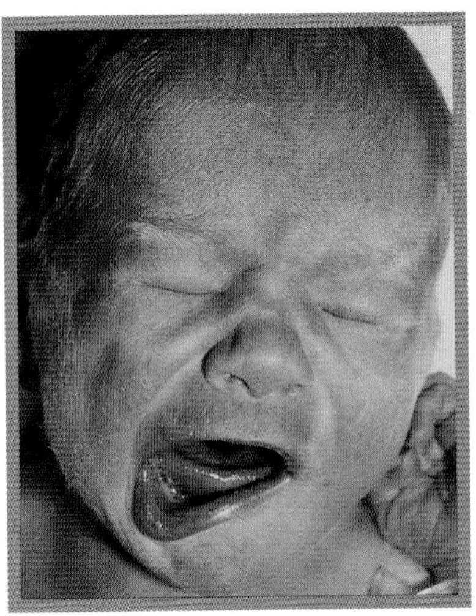

1.6 Facial palsy
This lower motor nerve palsy usually results from a forceps delivery during which pressure has been applied to the nerve as it exits the facial canal but it may also occur after local pressure *in utero* or during labour. Complete resolution is usual but a residual deficit may occur if the nerve fibres have been torn.

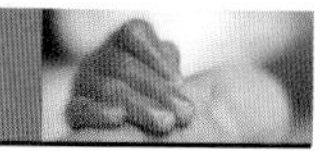

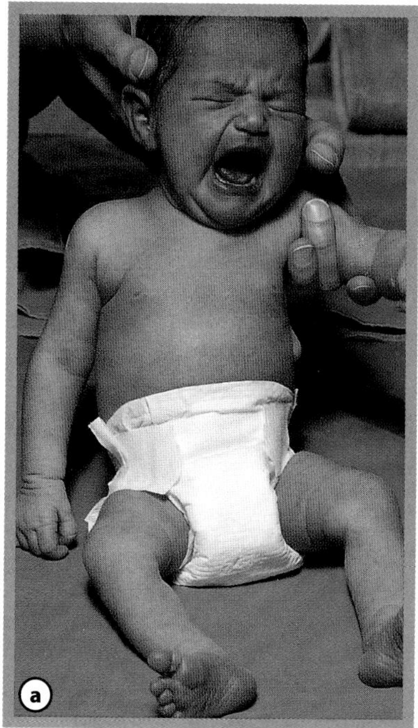

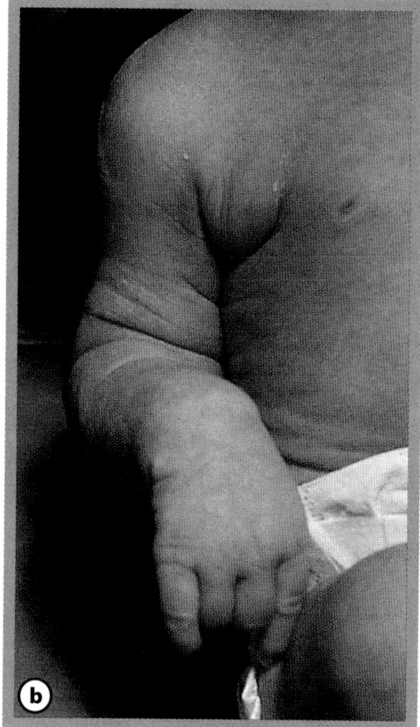

1.7a and 1.7b Erb's palsy

This may follow a traumatic delivery or shoulder presentation and represents a lesion of C5/6, resulting in adduction and internal rotation of the arm, with pronation of the forearm as shown. Hand power is usually retained. A full recovery may occur with physiotherapy, although some permanent deficit is more common.

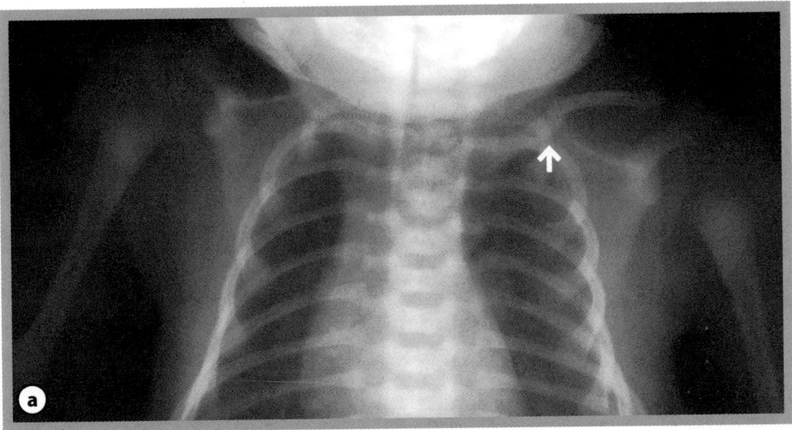

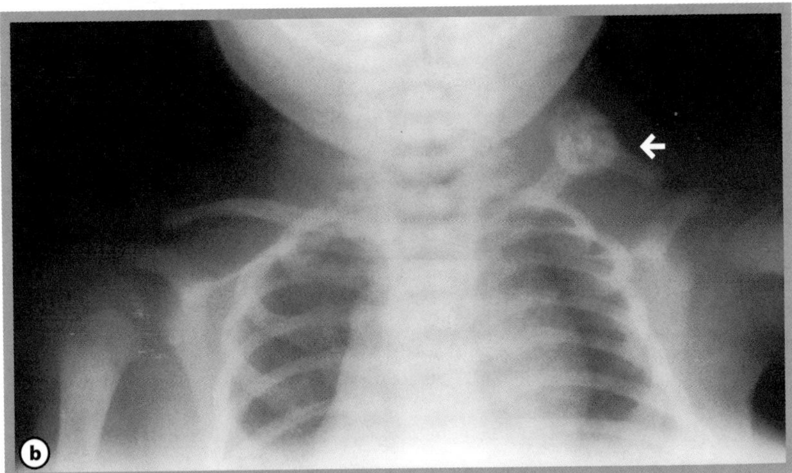

1.8a and 1.8b Fractured clavicle
This infant (1.8a) was born with shoulder dystocia. After birth the child was noted to be tachypnoeic; a routine radiograph revealed a left clavicular fracture. At the age of 2 weeks (1.8b), a fracture is evident with extensive callus formation involving the outer one-third of the right clavicle. Traumatic delivery, particularly resulting from a shoulder or breech presentation may cause this injury. Despite what may appear to be a very displaced fracture, complete union without residual bony deformity is the usual outcome.

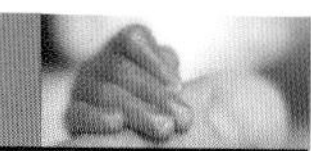

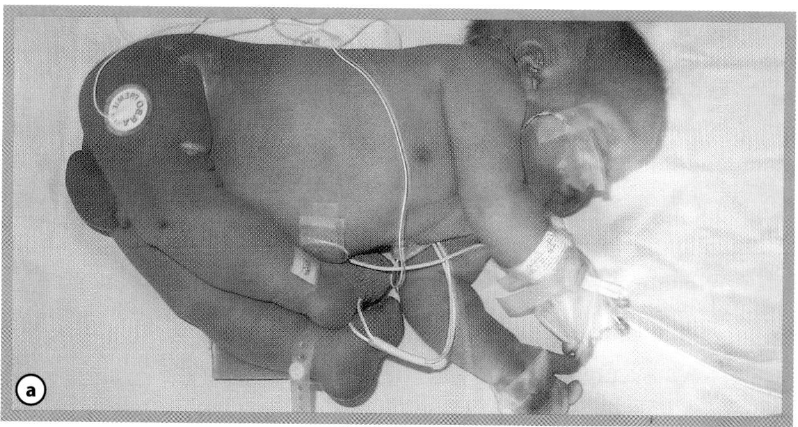

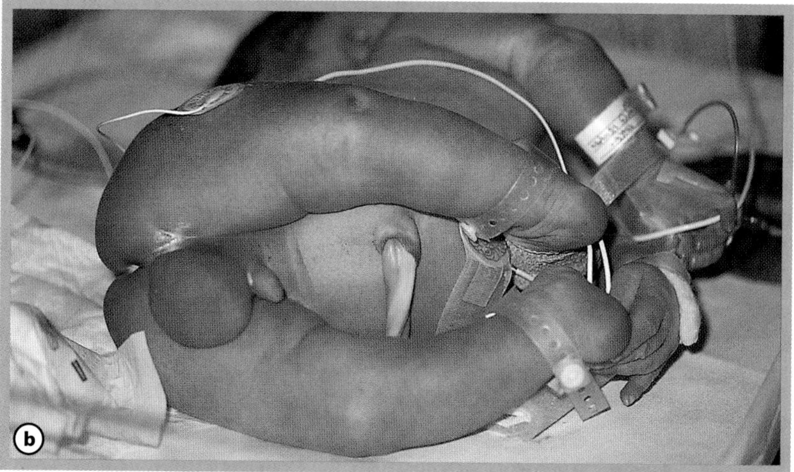

1.9a and 1.9b Breech hips
A marked positional abnormality of both hips is shown associated with bruising of the thighs after an extended breech delivery. Congenital dislocation of the hip is more common in infants born via breech. Even when infants have turned before delivery, they should be screened for congenital dislocation of the hip. Clinical examination in the first 24 hours will often exhibit instability of breech hips, although subsequent examination may be normal.

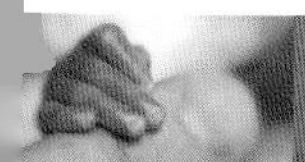

2 Skin/mucous membrane disorders

2.1a and 2.1b Milia

This common condition presents as numerous tiny white or yellow papules within the first few days. The lesions represent superficial epidermal cysts that occur particularly over the face and resolve spontaneously.

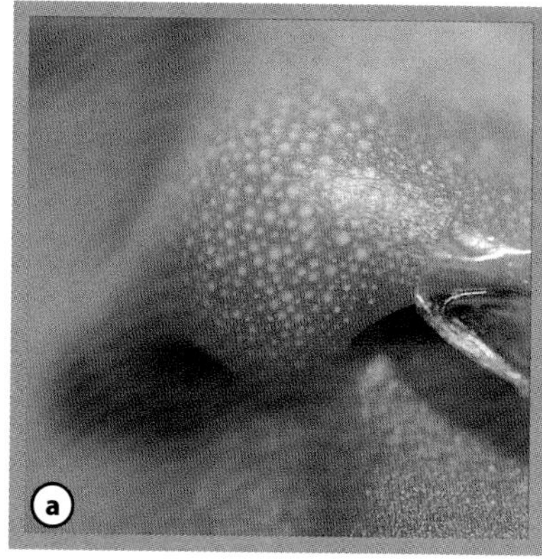

a

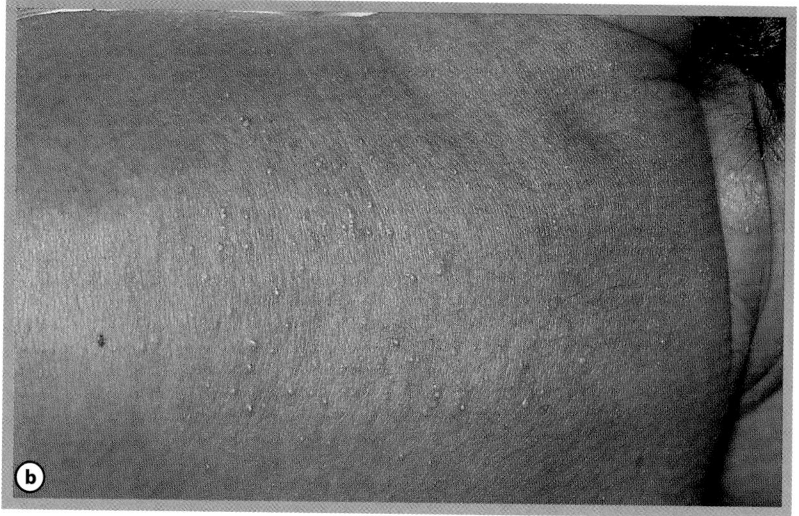

b

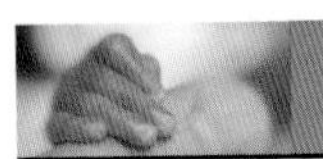

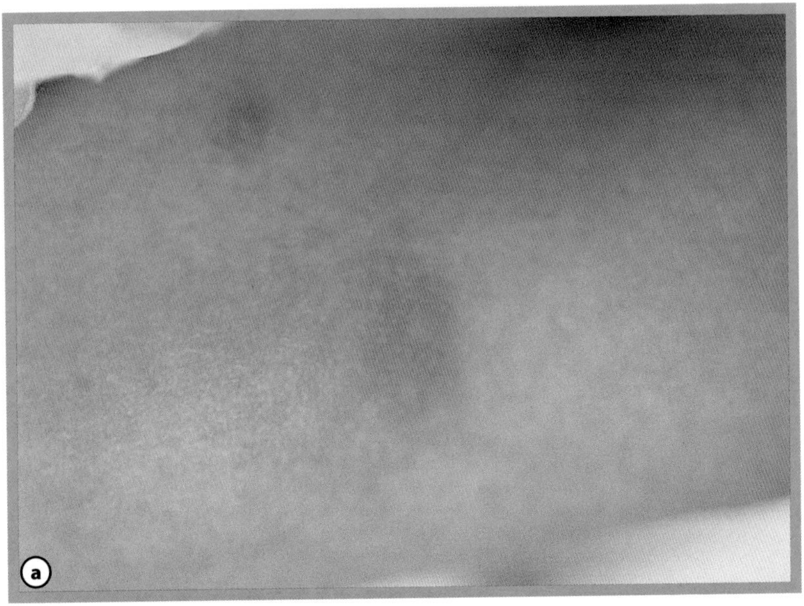

a

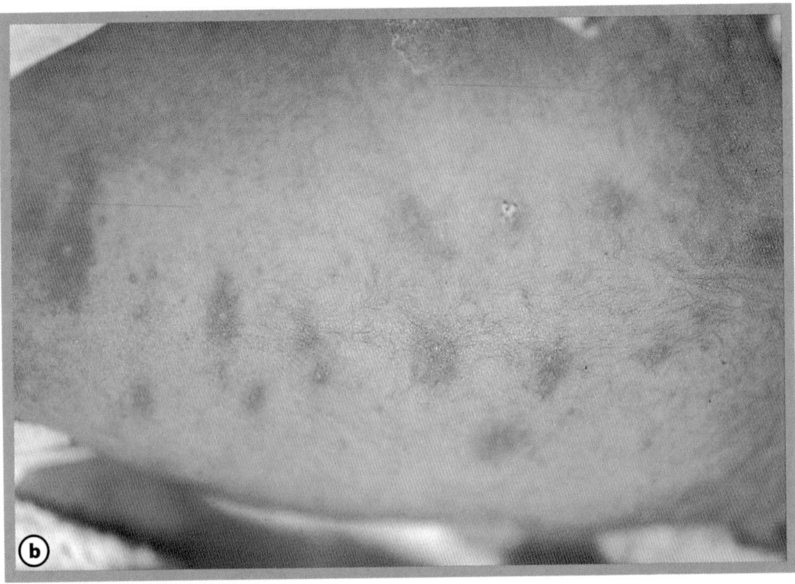

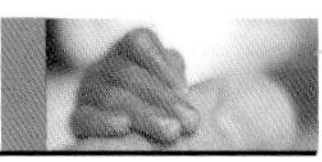

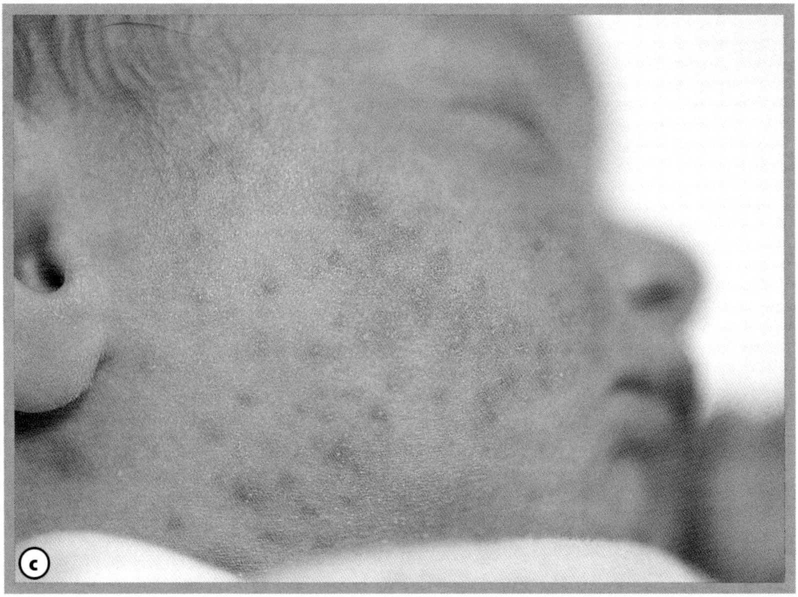

2.2a, 2.2b and 2.2c Erythema toxicum
This extremely common condition presents as yellow pustules on an erythematous base. There is extensive eosinophilia on histology but the cause is unknown. The condition resolves without treatment and antibiotics are not required. Confusion can arise between this and staphylococcal skin sepsis.

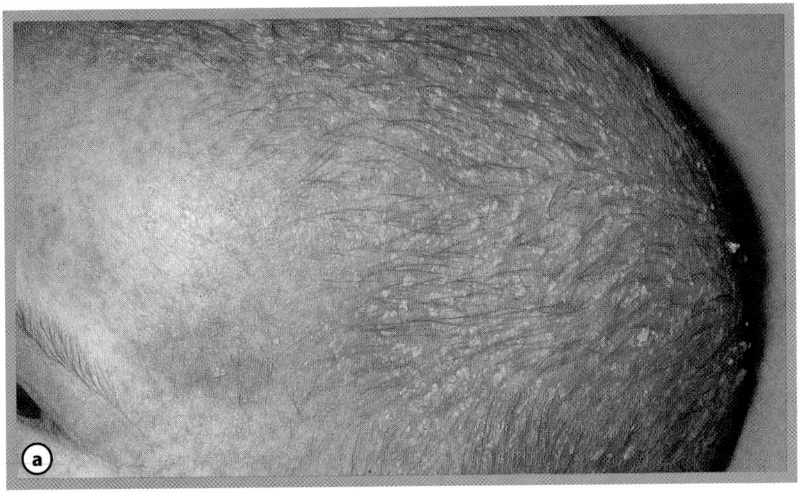

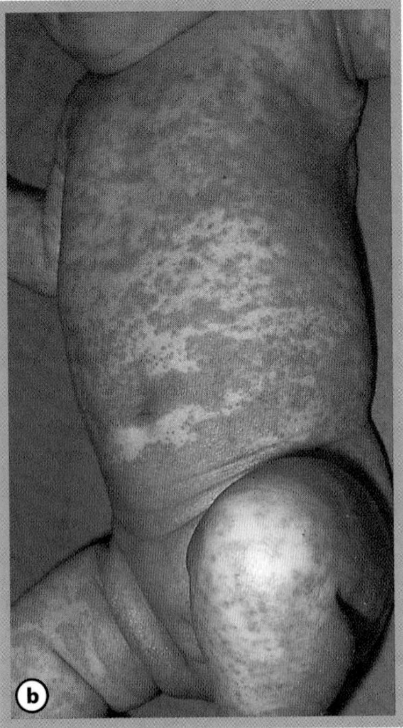

2.3a and 2.3b Seborrhoeic dermatitis
This condition, which may be indistinguishable from infantile eczema, is associated with erythema and scaling, particularly of the scalp, face and nappy area. Bacterial or fungal superinfection may occur. Treatment consists of emollient therapy and oil for the scalp. Steroids may be required for more inflamed areas and an antifungal topical agent may also be needed when candida is thought also to be present (see 2.4a and 2.4b).

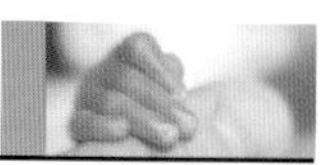

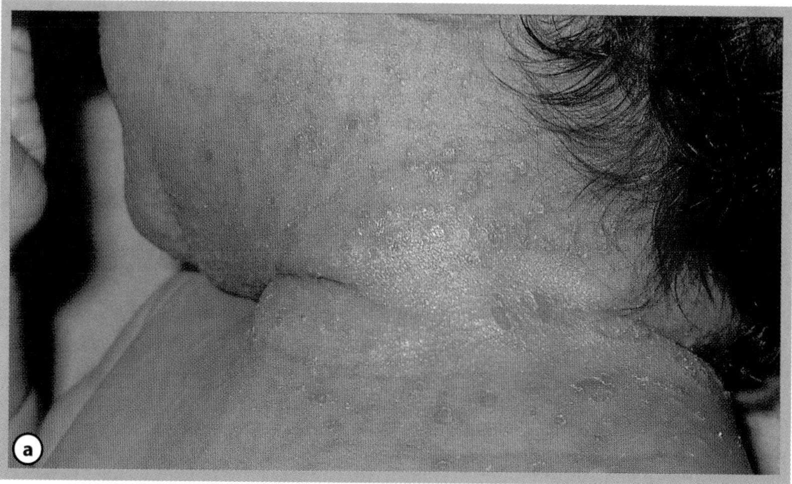

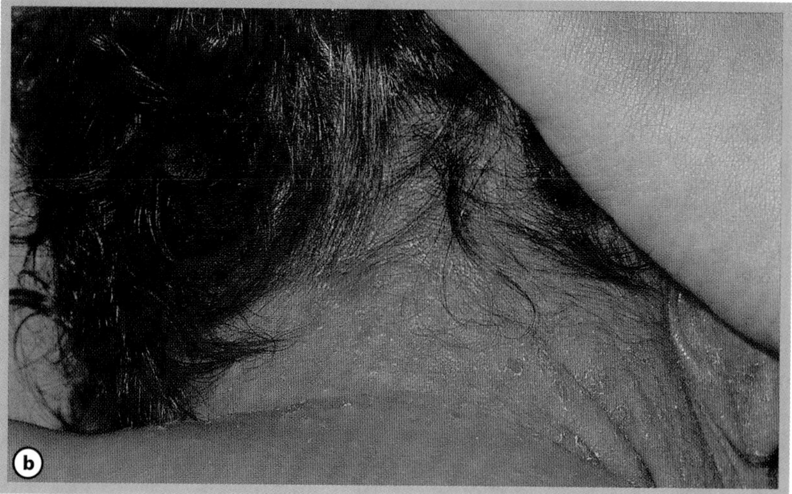

2.4a and 2.4b Seborrhoeic dermatitis with candida infection
A co-existent candida infection is present in this infant with symmetrical pustules apparent. Complete resolution occurred within 5 days of treatment with a combined antifungal and steroid preparation.

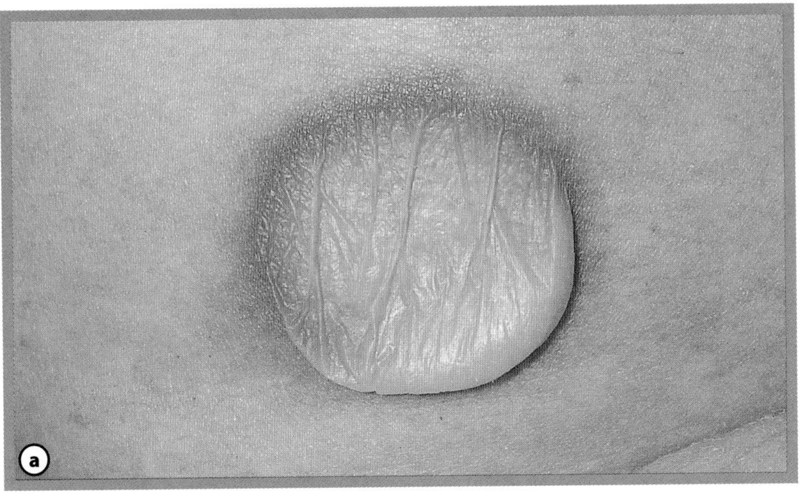

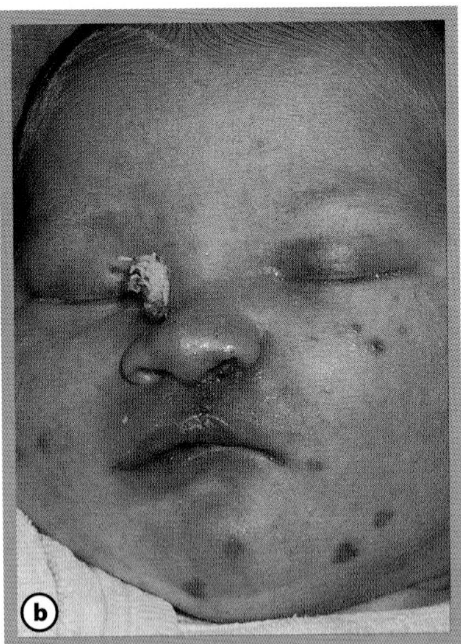

2.5a, 2.5b, 2.5c and 2.5d Staphylococcal skin sepsis
Staphylococcal skin infections in neonates may present as isolated pustules, cellulitis or paronychia. In this infant numerous lesions are seen, including an extensive area of infection around the inner canthus of the right eye, a paronychia of the ring finger and an area of cellulitis surrounding the fourth toe. Systemic flucloxacillin therapy is required.

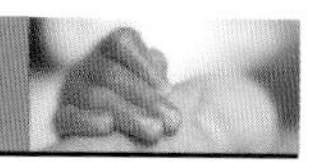

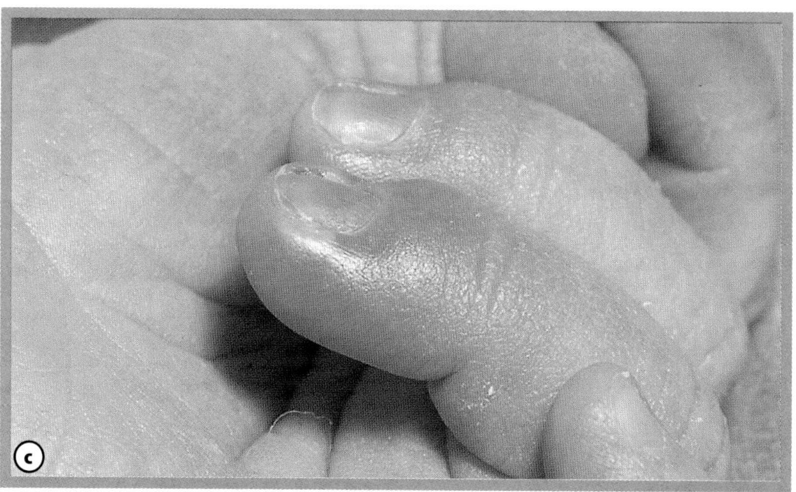
c

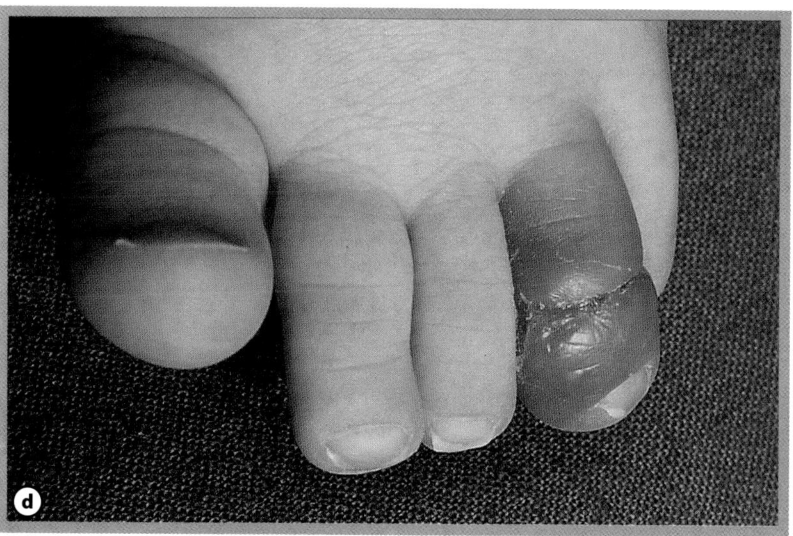
d

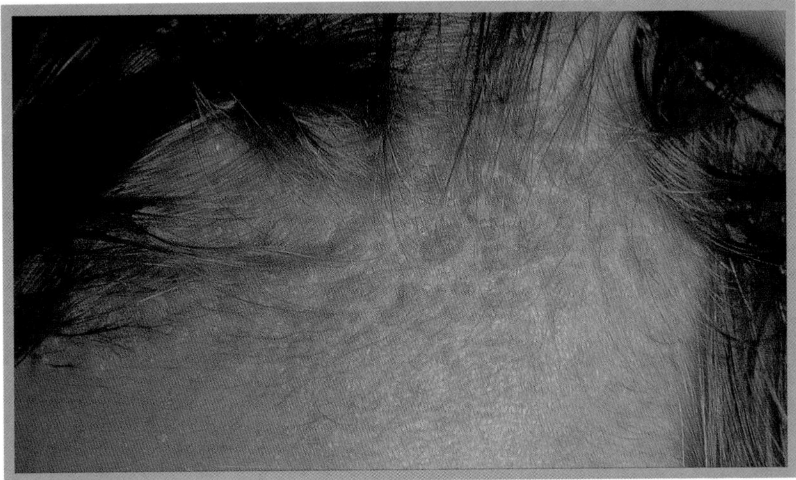

2.6 Cradle cap

Cradle cap may occur in isolation or as part of seborrhoeic dermatitis and is characterized by scaling of the scalp. Treatment is with oil preparations such as arachis oil.

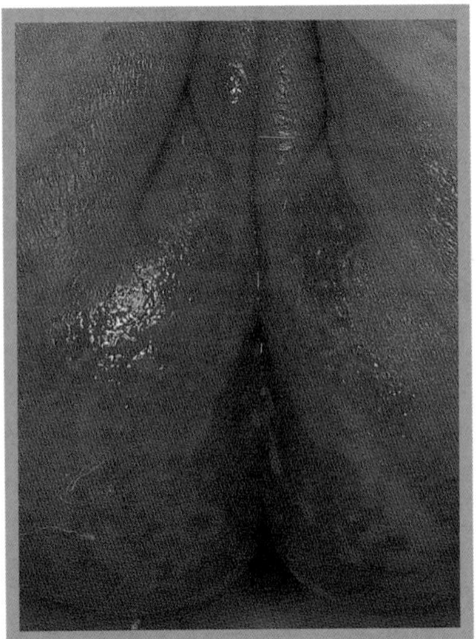

2.7 Perineal candidiasis

Candidiasis is one of the common nappy rashes, although it may be difficult to distinguish from other common causes, including seborrhoeic dermatitis, infantile eczema and ammoniacal dermatitis on which candidiasis is often superimposed. In its pure form the presence of satellite lesions and the absence of lesions in the skin folds suggests *Candida*. Treatment consists of topical antifungal agents which in practice are often used in combination with a steroid preparation.

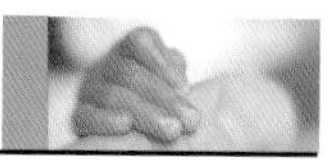

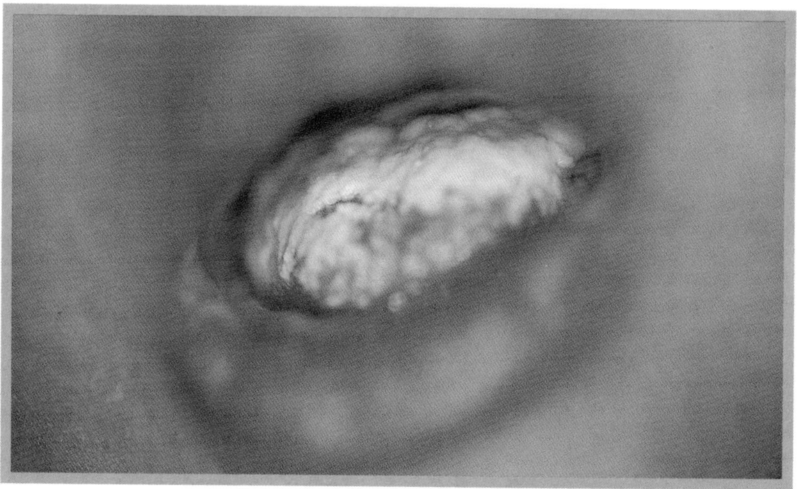

2.8 Oral candidiasis

Oral candidiasis presents as white plaques on the tongue or buccal mucus and may, if severe, lead to bleeding and poor feeding. Treatment consists of oral antifungal agents. It is important that all teats are cleaned between use as they may provide a source for persisting infection.

2.9 Mucous retention cyst

Infants are sometimes born with a mucous retention cyst. This can be frightening for the parents who should, however, be reassured that these cysts are totally benign and transient.

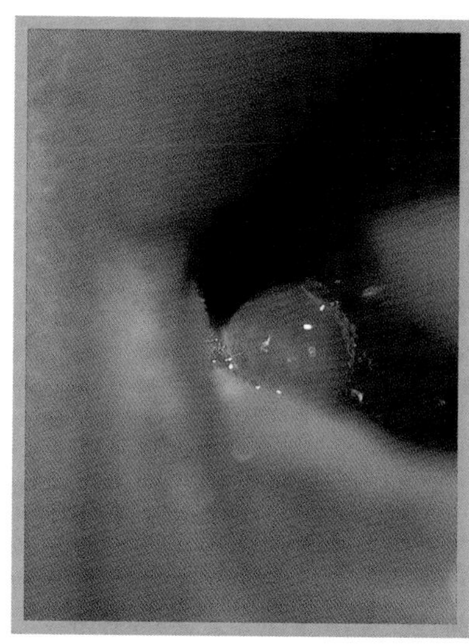

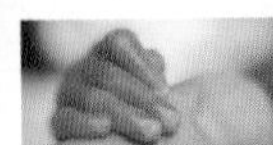

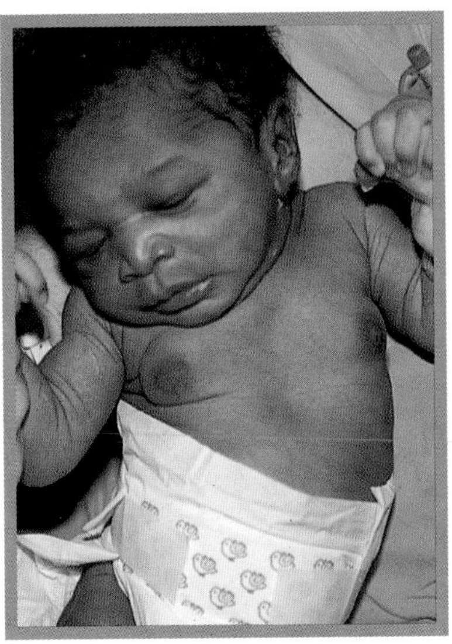

2.10 Gynaecomastia

Breast engorgement occurs not infrequently following birth. It is caused by the presence of maternal hormones and is usually transient. Occasionally antibiotic treatment is required if an abscess develops (*see* **3.6**).

3 Miscellaneous

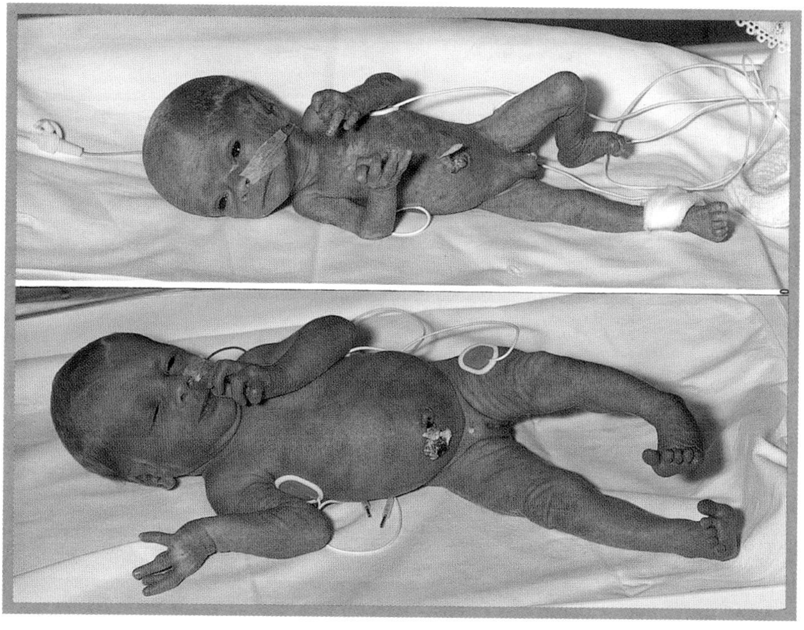

3.1 Twin to twin transfusion syndrome

An imbalance in perfusion within a monochorionic placenta resulted in growth retardation of one and polycythaemia of the other twin. Note the spared head growth in the smaller twin and the plethora of the larger twin. Clinical problems are often more severe in the recipient with complications of polycythaemia, for example, jaundice, thrombocytopaenia, cerebral infarct and necrotizing enterocolitis.

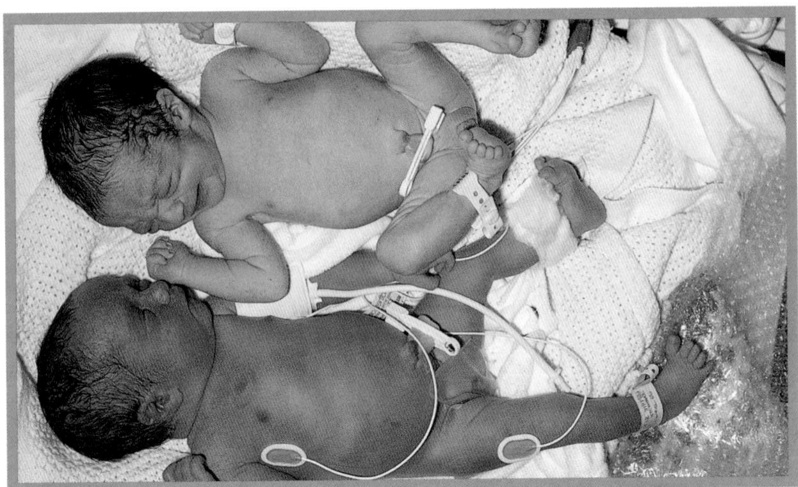

3.2 Acute fetofetal transfusion

An acute transfer of blood occurred between these twins with one born anaemic and the other polycythaemic. Urgent transfusion of the anaemic infant is required; a partial exchange of the recipient twin is needed if symptomatic with a packed cell volume of greater than 60% or if asymptomatic with a packed cell volume greater than 65–70%. The exact packed cell volume at which an exchange transfusion is indicated is hotly debated with some long-term studies showing no adverse effects of untreated asymptomatic polycythaemia. Most authorities would agree however that a packed cell volume of greater than 70% is an absolute indication for an exchange transfusion.

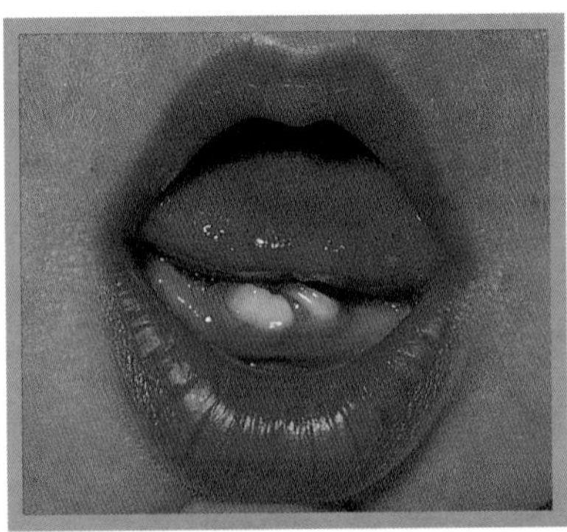

3.3 Neonatal teeth

These are rare and may either be present at birth or erupt within the first month of life. These teeth are often loose and should be removed.

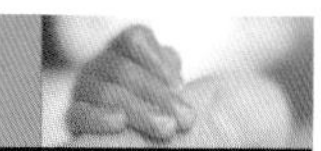

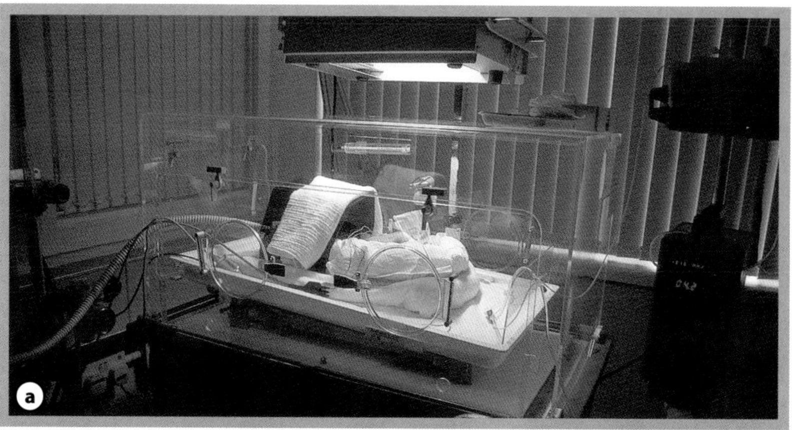

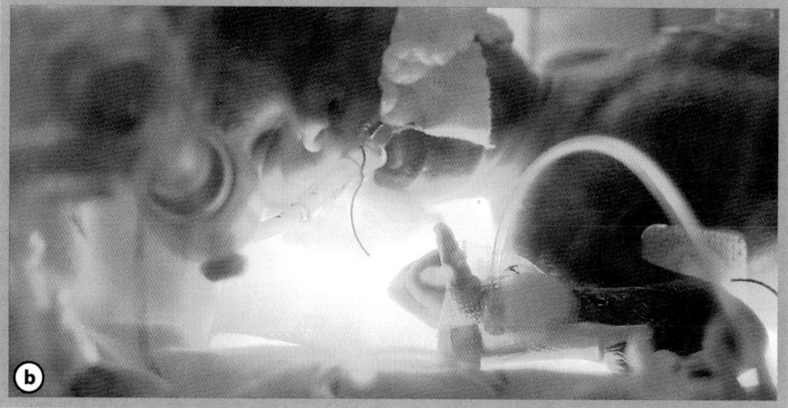

3.4a and 3.4b Jaundice

Jaundice is one of the most common neonatal problems in the term infant. It is usually physiological in nature but other causes (e.g. haemolysis and sepsis) should be considered. In breast-fed babies, early jaundice is often the result of poor feeding, with dehydration exacerbating physiological jaundice, as opposed to any effect of breast milk itself at that stage. Persisting unconjugated jaundice should prompt a search for causes such as hypothyroidism, glucose-6-phosphate dehydrogenase deficiency, galactosaemia and sepsis (e.g. urinary tract infection). Two types of phototherapy are shown, above and below the infant.

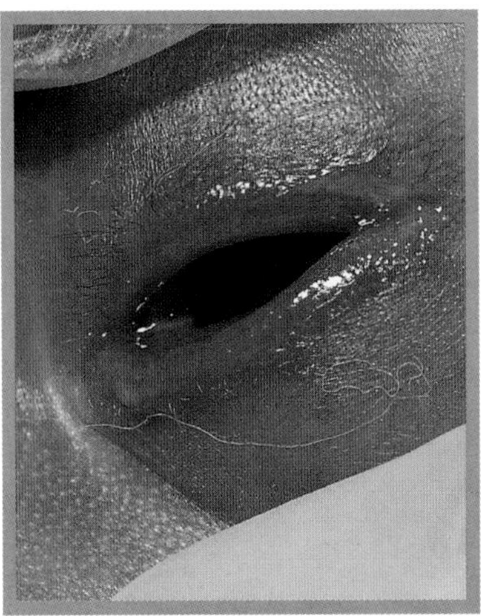

3.5 Conjunctivitis

Neonatal conjunctivitis is common and often bilateral. Swabs should be taken before starting antibiotic drops and neomycin is an appropriate first-line therapy. Chloramphenicol if used initially may affect later swabs for *Chlamydia* by inhibiting its growth on culture. A persisting infection should raise the suspicion of *Chlamydia* and culture and enzyme immunofluorescence assay swabs should be taken. Treatment for *Chlamydia* is oral erythromycin for 2 weeks, both to clear the conjunctivitis and to reduce the risk of associated pneumonia.

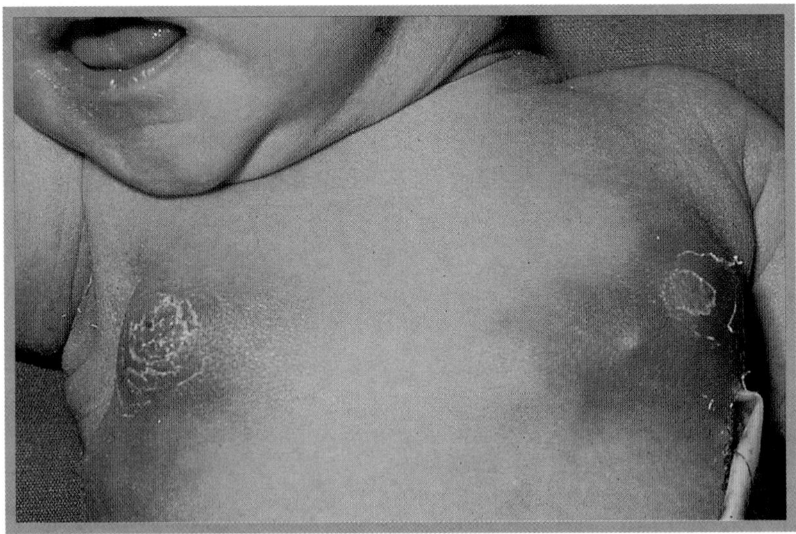

3.6 Mastitis

This infant demonstrates redness and swelling of both breasts, reflecting infection complicating gynaecomastia (*see* **2.10**).

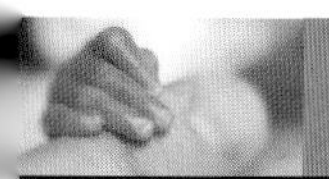

4 Skin

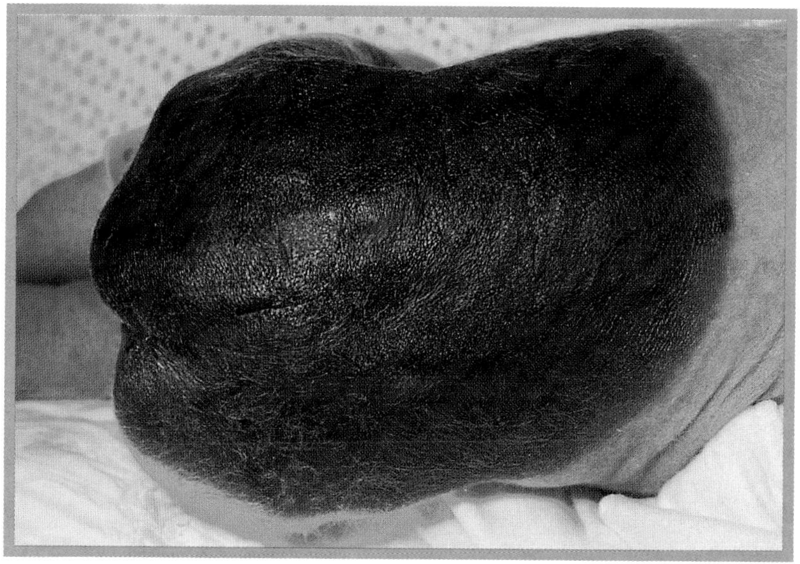

4.1 Giant congenital melanocytic naevus (bathing trunk type)
This extensive naevus is called bathing trunk naevus because of its characteristic distribution. Like the similar localized melanocytic naevi (*see* **4.2**), the risk of malignant change is not as high as previously thought. Treatment is for cosmetic reasons and consists initially of removal of the epidermal layer within the first few weeks of life. The skin is shaved off but caution is needed to ensure the dermal layer is not removed because this would lead to scarring.

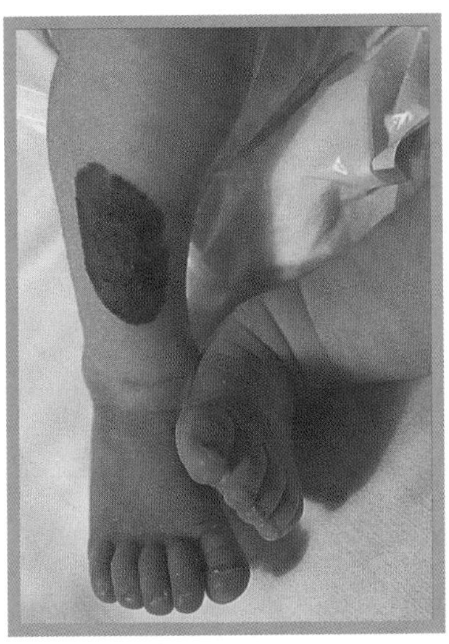

4.2 Congenital melanocytic naevus

This naevus has a classic raised, dark and hairy appearance. Treatment of smaller lesions is by complete excision. There is a slightly increased risk of ultimate malignant change in these lesions.

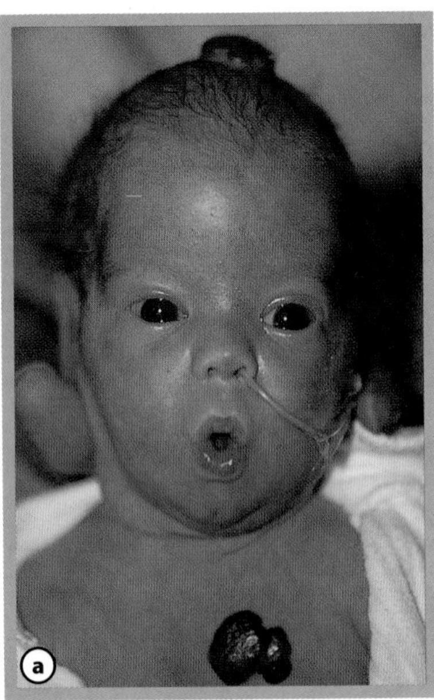

4.3a, 4.3b and 4.3c Strawberry naevi

This ex-preterm infant has two extensive strawberry naevi. These cavernous haemangiomas represent clusters of angiogenetic cells and usually increase in size over the first 12 months. However, the vast majority ultimately regress. Complications include haemorrhage and infection; if sited precariously naevi, may interfere with vital functions (e.g. vision, *see* **4.4**).

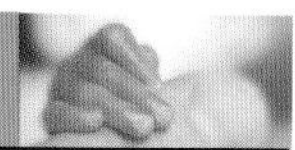

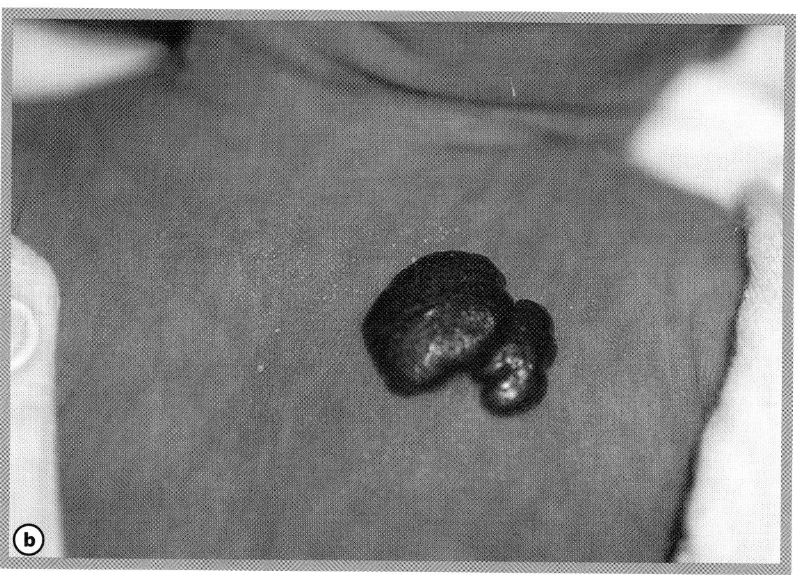
b

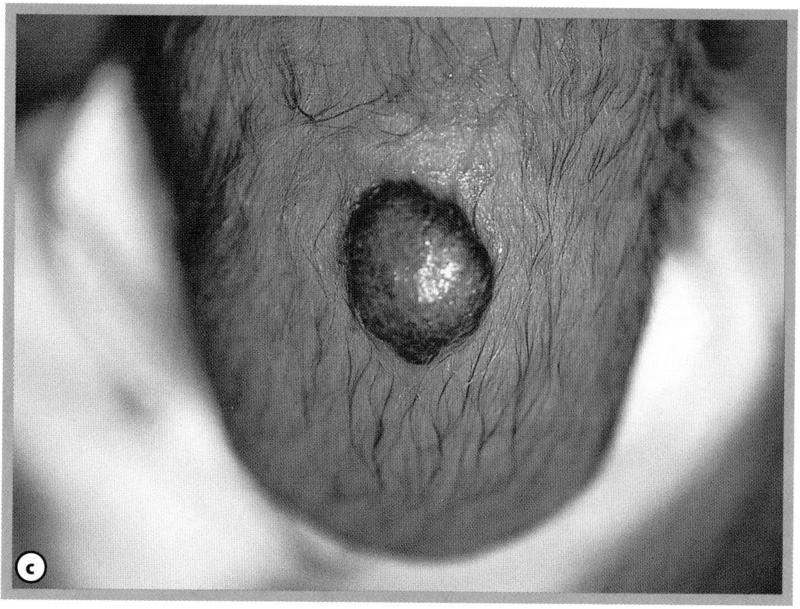

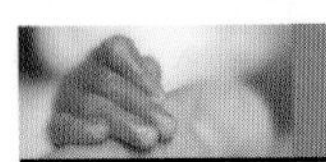

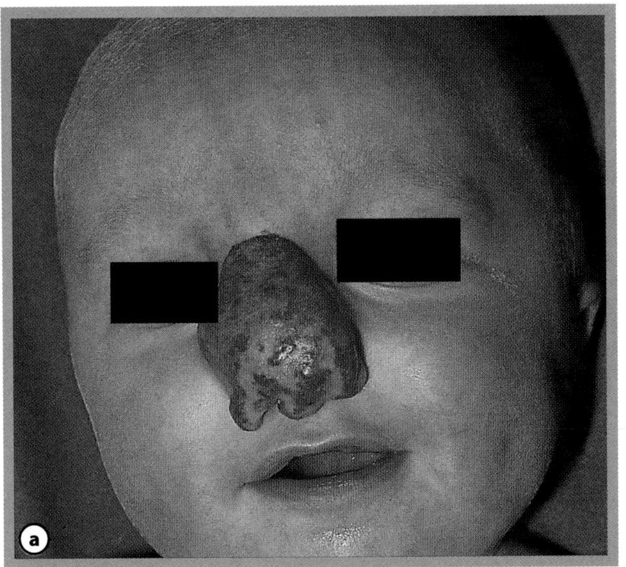
a

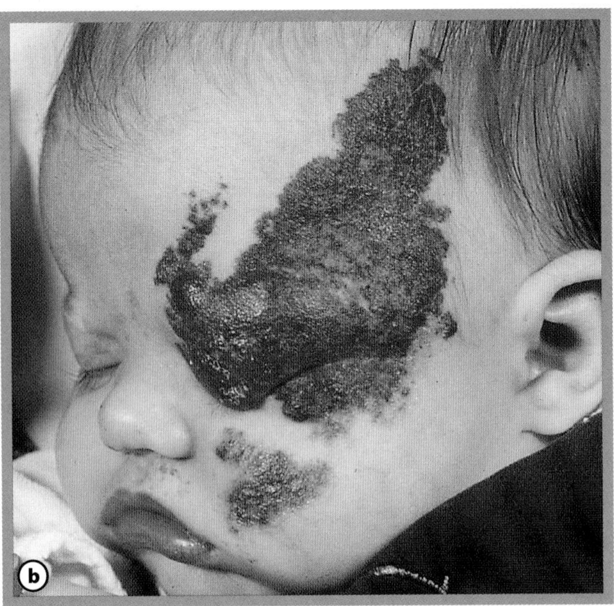
b

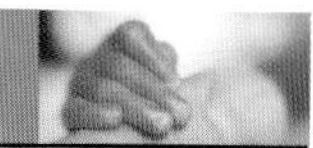

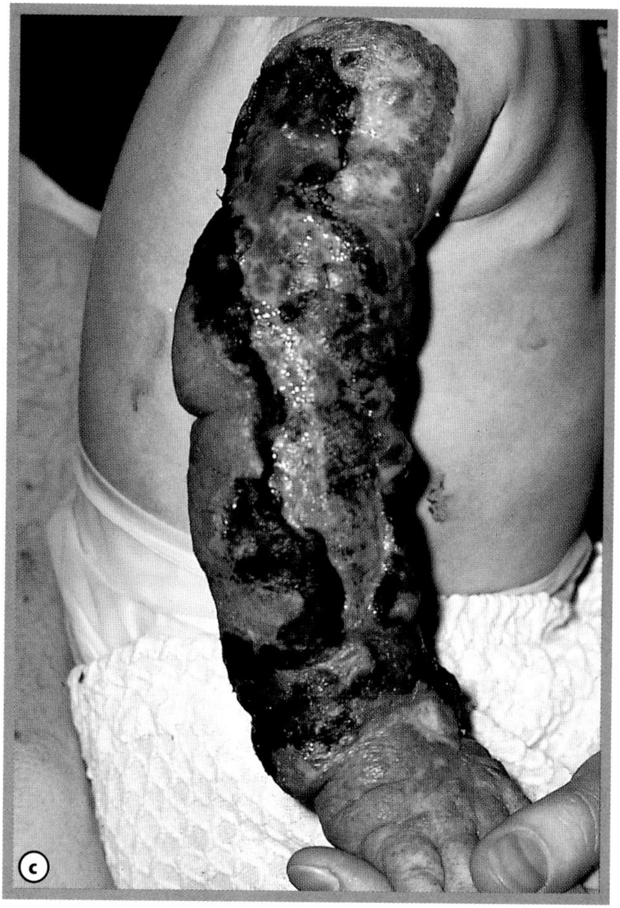

4.4a, 4.4b and 4.4c Extensive haemangiomas

These pictures show the potential complications of extensive haemangiomas, affecting the vital functions of smell (**4.2a**) and vision (**4.4b**) and causing infection and skin breakdown (**4.2c**). In **4.4c**, the haemangioma encircles the entire arm and the skin has ulcerated with a resultant wide area of skin loss, similar to a full-thickness burn. Very large naevi may be associated with thrombocytopenia, known as Kasabach–Merritt syndrome.

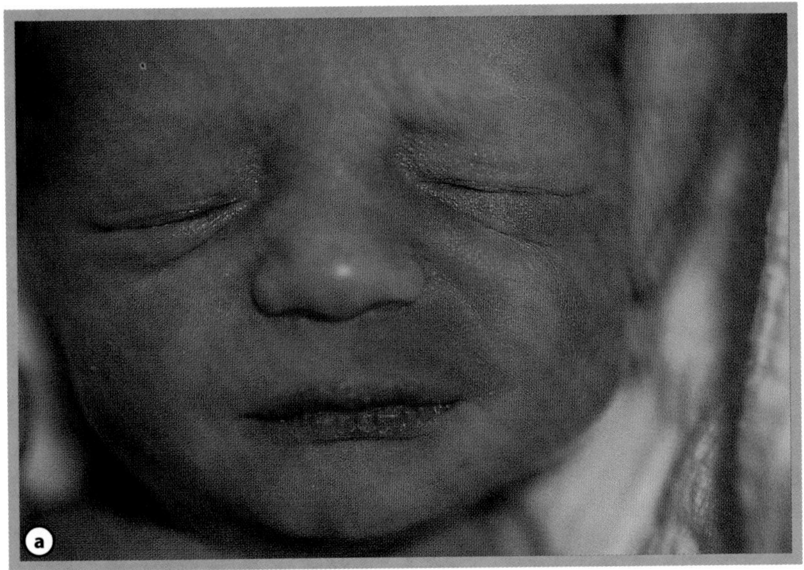
a

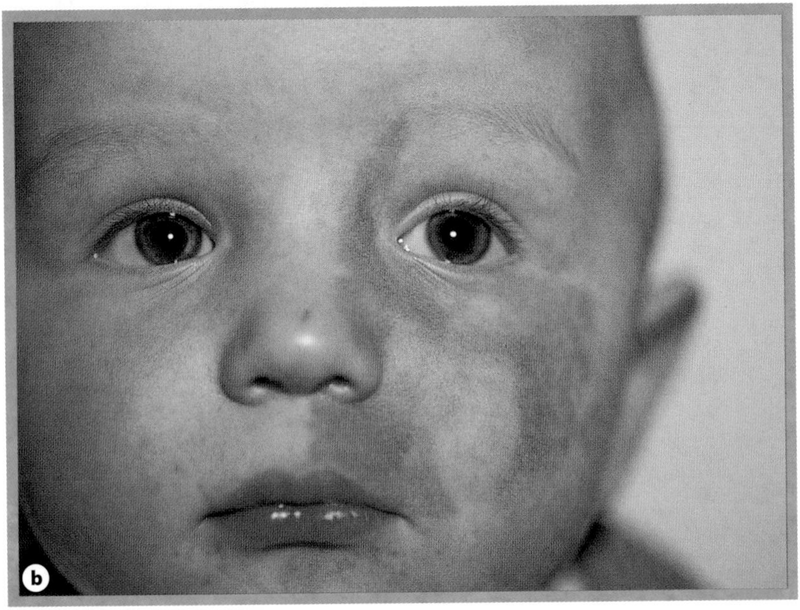

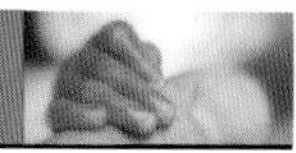

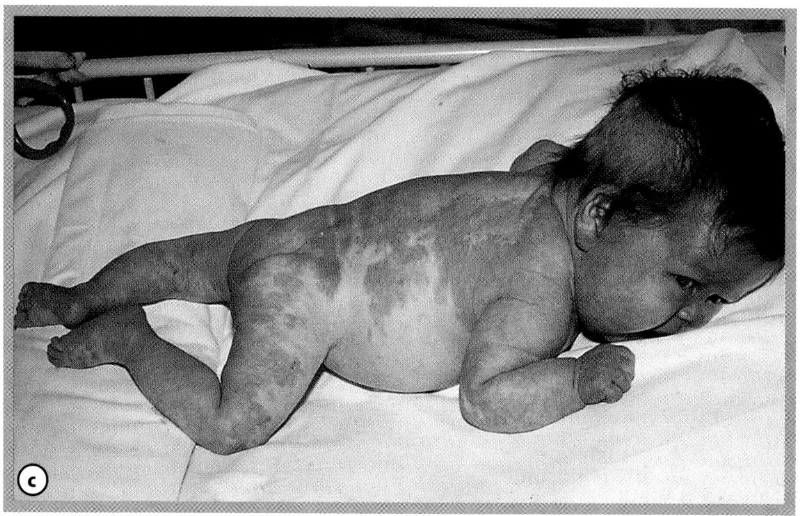

4.5a, 4.5b and 4.5c Port wine stain
Unlike strawberry naevi, these capillary haemangiomas persist and darken with age. They have a particular predilection for the face (**4.5a** at birth, **4.5b** 9 months later) and back of neck, although they may be very extensive (**4.5c**). Port wine stains may be associated with intra-cranial vascular anomalies (in Sturge–Weber syndrome) and limb hypertrophy (in Klippel–Trenaunay syndrome). Laser therapy is now established as an effective cosmetic treatment. In Sturge–Weber syndrome, severe physical and cognitive neurodisability may result, with associated intractable seizures.

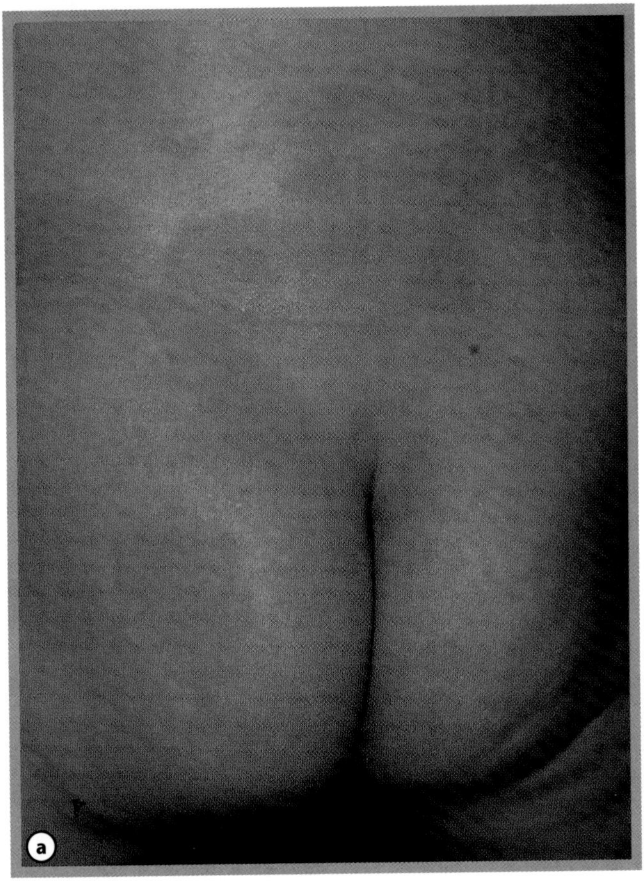

4.6a, 4.6b and 4.6c Blue spots

Congenital pigmented naevi known as blue spots are extremely common, particularly but not exclusively, in infants of black or Asian origin. The naevi occur most commonly over the sacral area and buttocks but may be present over the shoulders and legs and be extensive (**4.6b** and **4.6c**). Although they commonly fade over the first year of life, they may persist but there is no increased risk of malignancy.

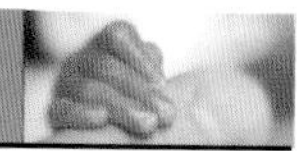

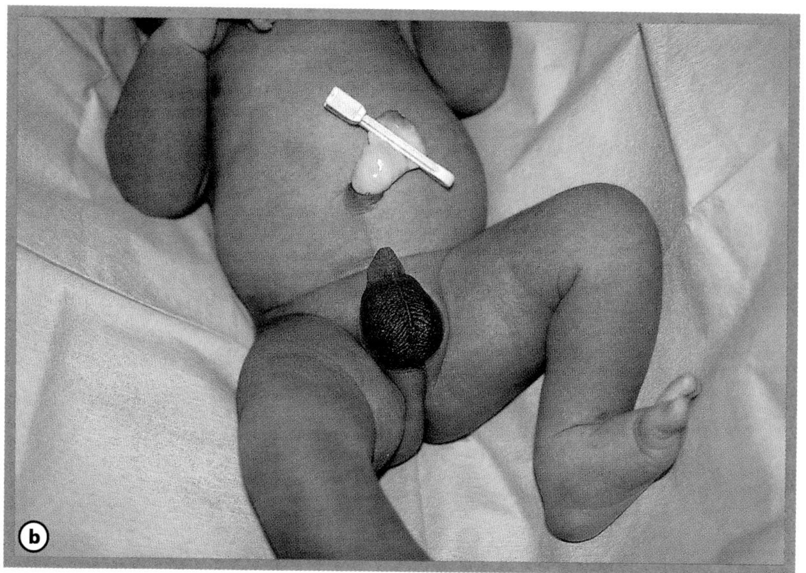

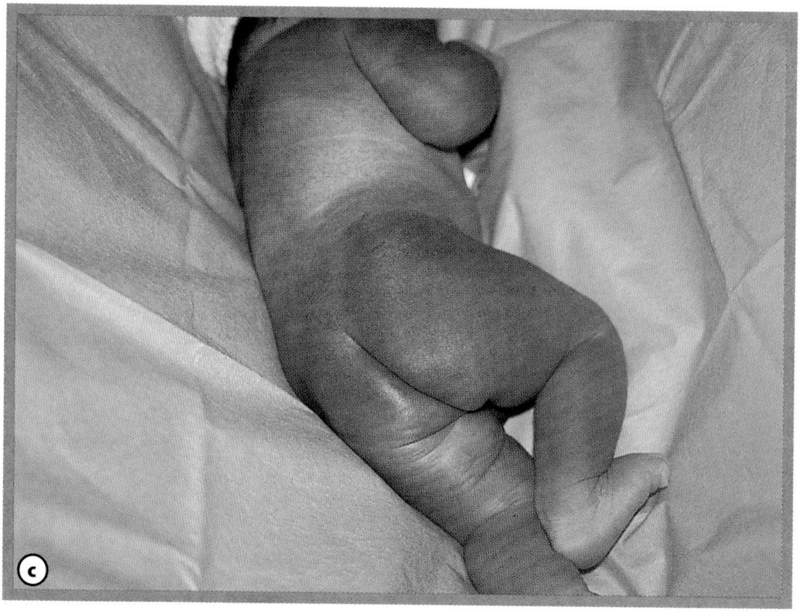

c

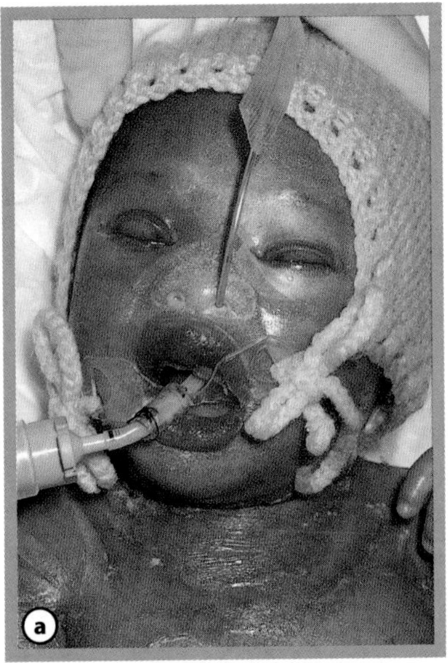

4.7a and 4.7b Collodion baby
The skin is bright red and tight and bilateral ectropion of the eyelids is apparent. The entire epidermal layer will shed within a few weeks and will reveal either normal skin beneath or more commonly an ichthyotic condition. The infant shown required ventilation for respiratory failure and ultimately died.

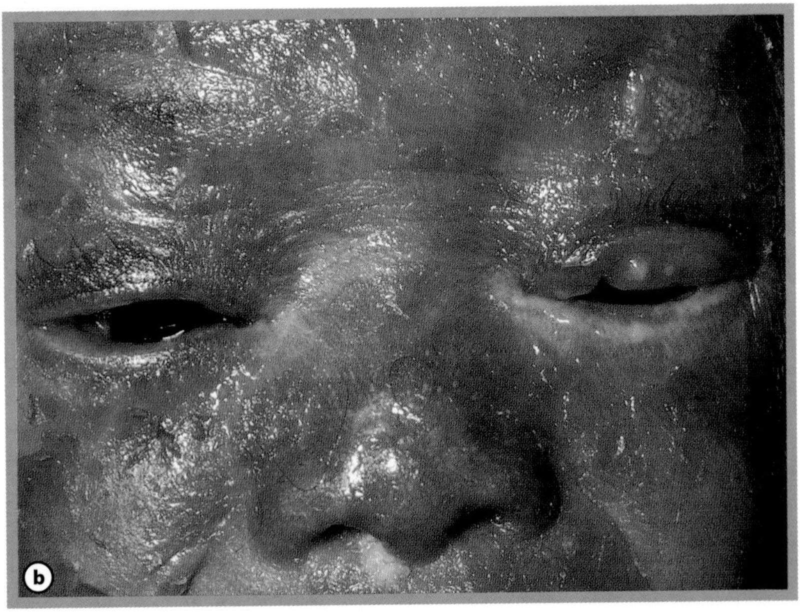

b

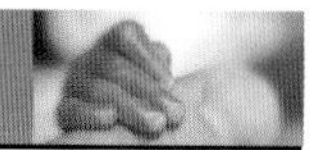

4.8 Epidermal naevus

This naevus is usually present at birth and is a raised plaque-like lesion that becomes papillomatous. It is significant in its association with other system abnormalities, e.g. central nervous system (seizures, learning disability, tumours), spinal and cardiac. When such an association occurs, the condition is called epidermal naevus syndrome.

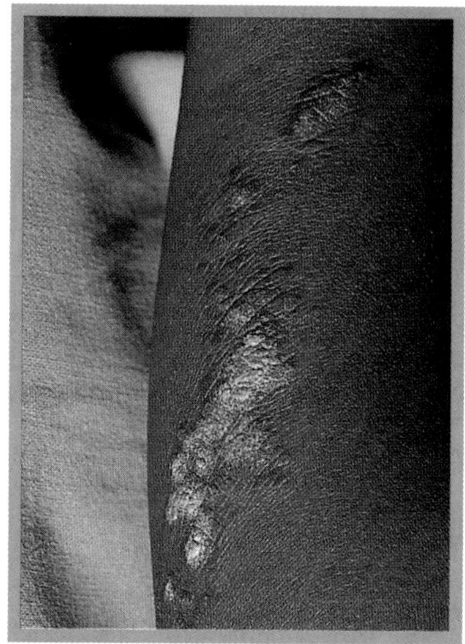

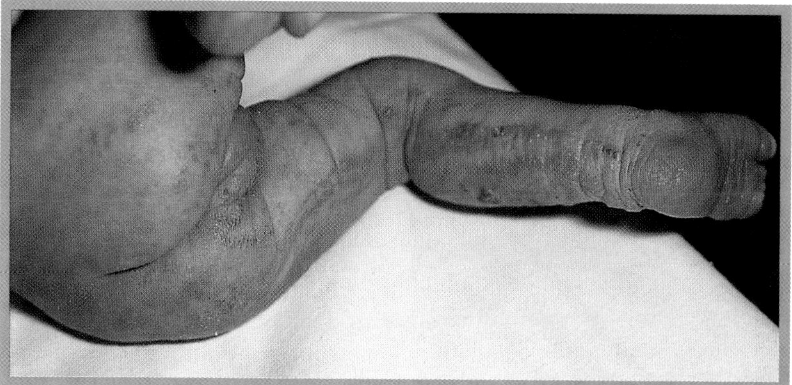

4.9 Incontinentia pigmenti

In this X-linked dominant condition, the lesions go through three distinct phases, commencing as an erythematous widespread linear rash, replaced within weeks by a verrucous phase and finally developing into the classical hyperpigmented streaky rash shown, which is said to follow the cleavage lines of Blashkow. The risk of intra-cranial pathology is high and the condition is usually fatal in boys *in utero*.

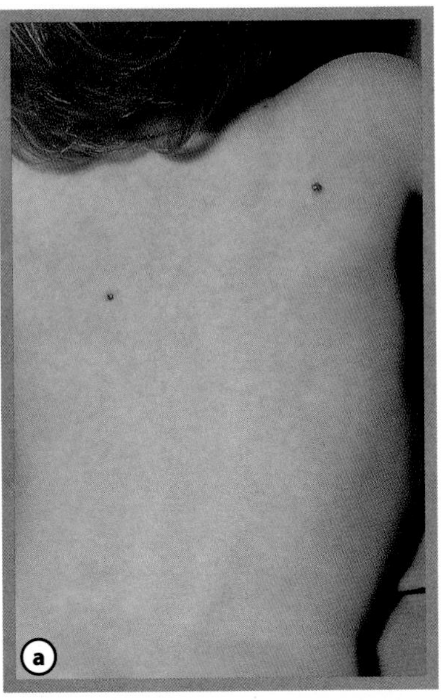

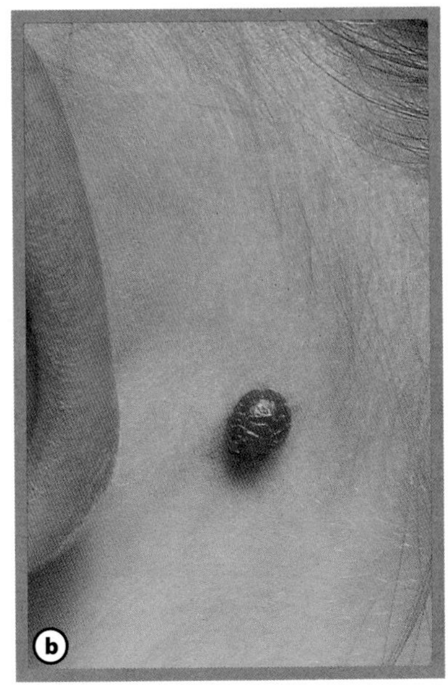

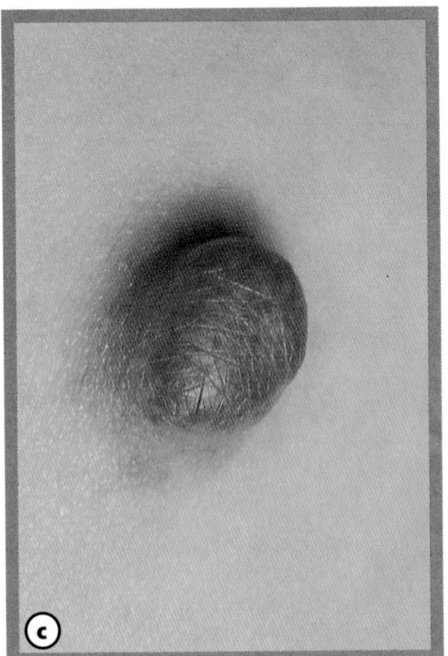

4.10a, 4.10b and 4.10c Disseminated haemangiomatosis

In this condition multiple haemangiomas occur and have the appearance (as shown) of small papular reddish-blue haemangiomas. Although the skin appearances are not striking, their importance relates to the associated underlying abnormalities relating to the presence of haemangiomas on vital organs, which may prove ultimately fatal.

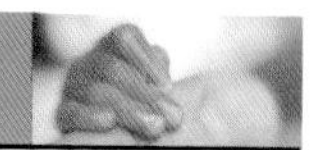

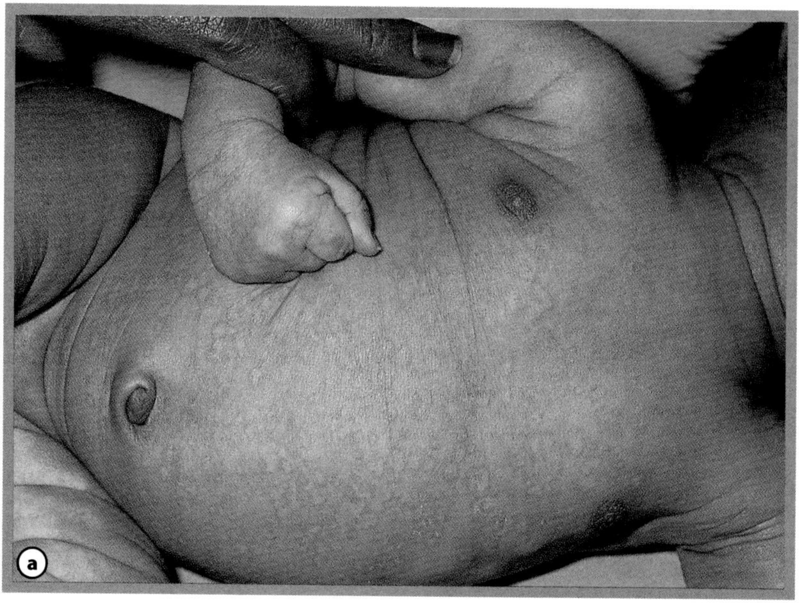

4.11a and 4.11b Annular erythema

This infant, born to a hepatitis B positive mother, presented at 2 weeks with an annular erythematous rash. A skin biopsy performed showed the characteristics of systemic lupus erythematosus. At 6 weeks of age, the infant was failing to thrive and presented with a pneumocystis pneumonia. He survived a prolonged ventilatory course and an unclassifiable, possibly transient T-cell mediated immunodeficiency was found. HIV serology was negative.

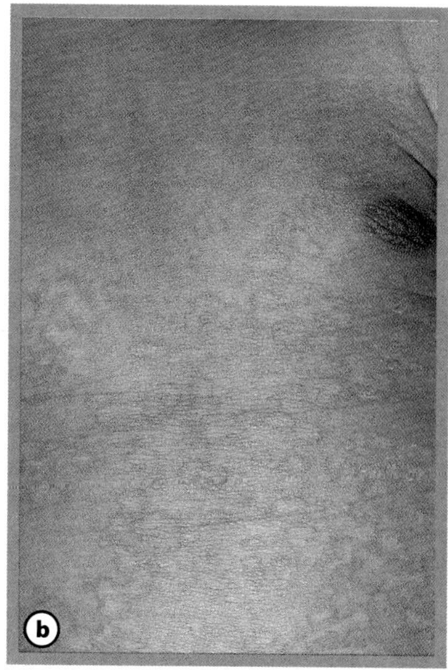

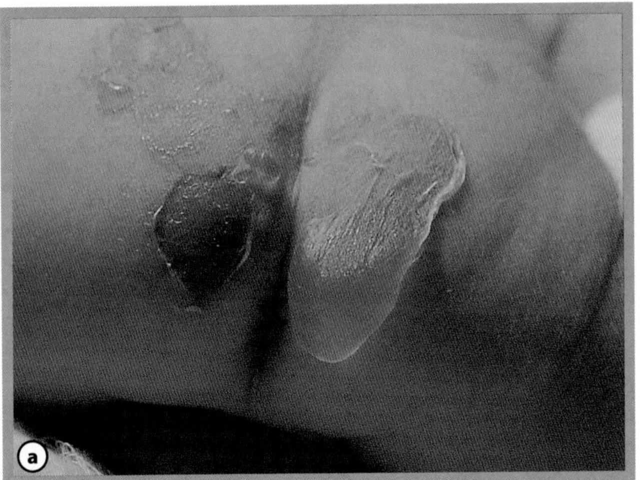

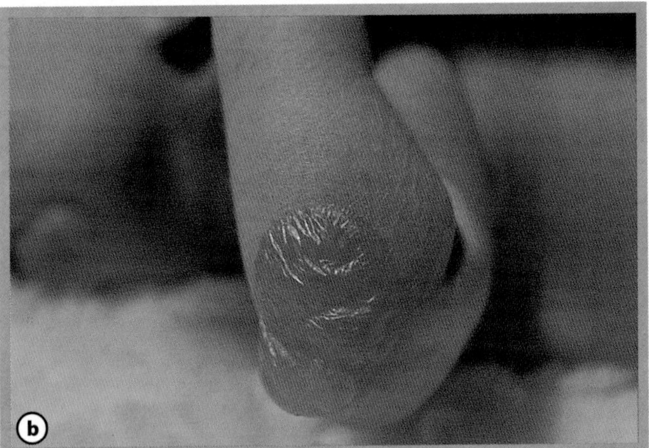

4.12a and 4.12b Epidermolysis bullosa
This is an autosomally inherited disorder. There are many different forms of the disease, the classification depending on the cleavage plane of the blister. The blisters are caused by minimal trauma, such as rubbing of the skin, or they may arise spontaneously. Depending on the type, healing may be complete or more commonly cause scarring.

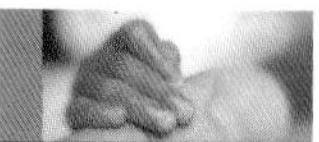

4.13 Toxic epidermal necrolysis

This has similar features to erythema multiforme and may represent the severe end of the disease spectrum. Generalized erythema with desquamating bullae and involvement of the conjunctiva and oral mucosa occurs. Severe systemic upset is associated. In neonates the most likely cause is infection. Treatment is supportive with broad-spectrum intra-venous antibiotics.

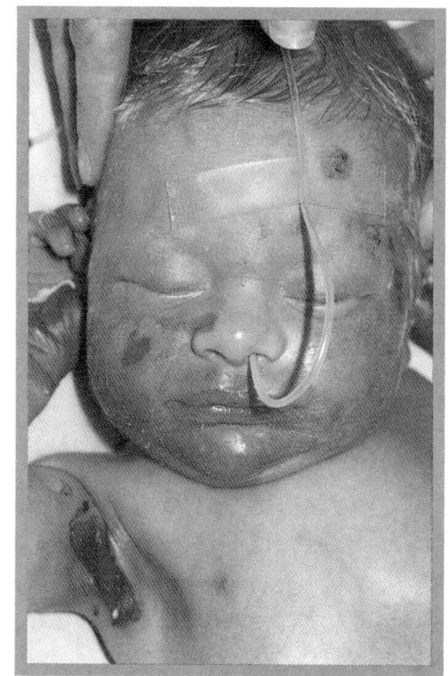

4.14 Neonatal lupus syndrome

This infant shows the classical facial butterfly rash of lupus. The neonatal lupus syndrome is associated with the passage of maternal anti-Ro antibodies across the placenta. The condition is associated with increased risk of spontaneous miscarriage, neonatal heart block, thrombocytopaenia and hepatosplenomegaly. Spontaneous resolution occurs as the maternal antibodies clear.

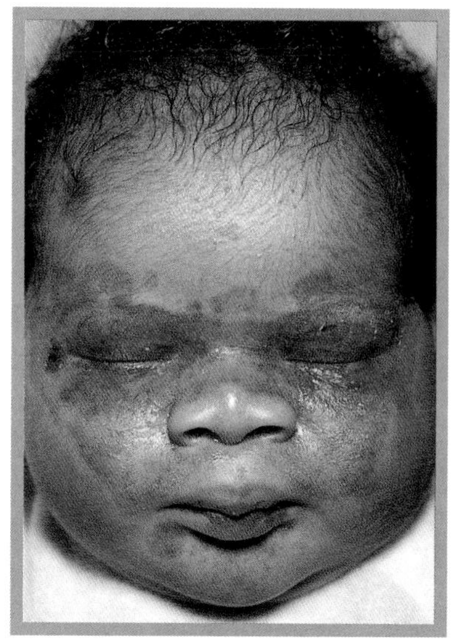

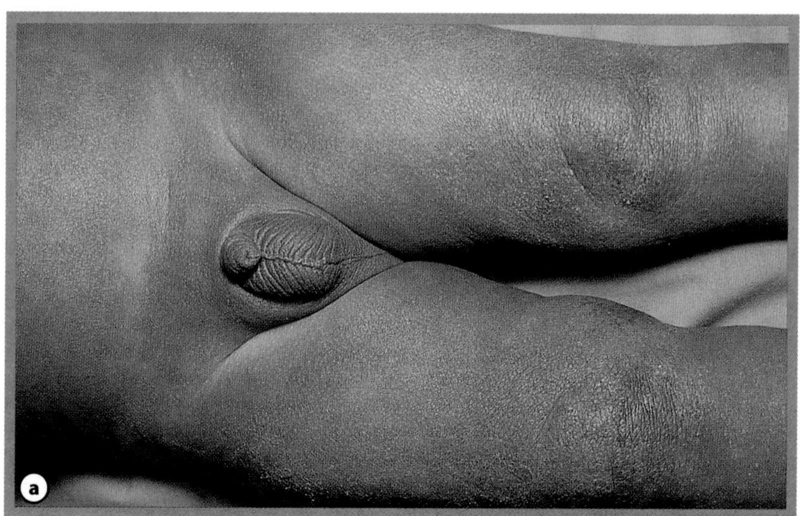

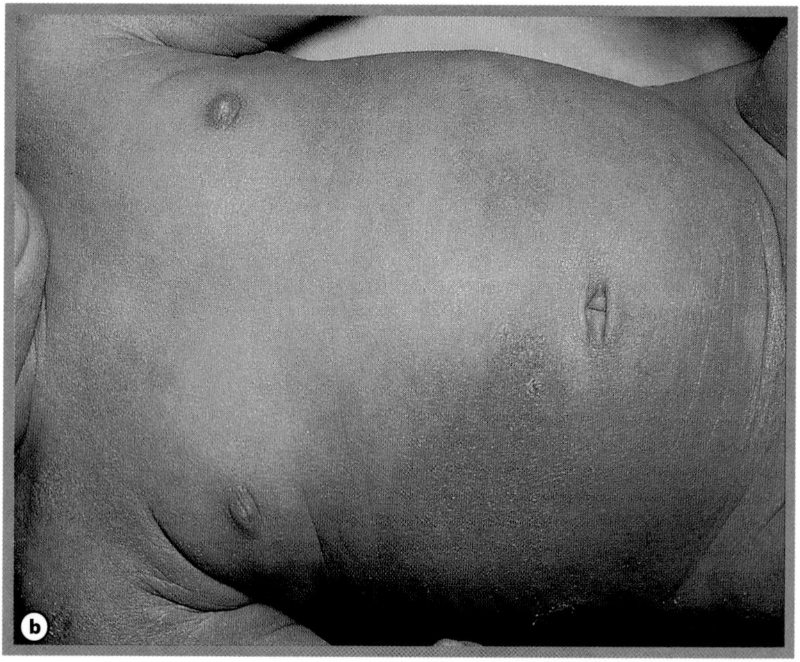

b

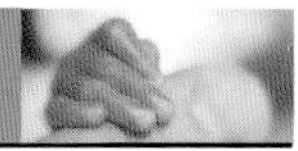

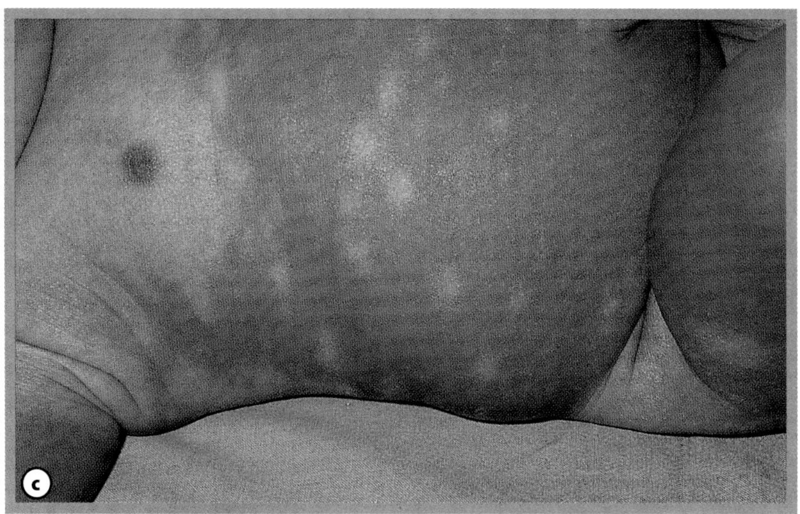

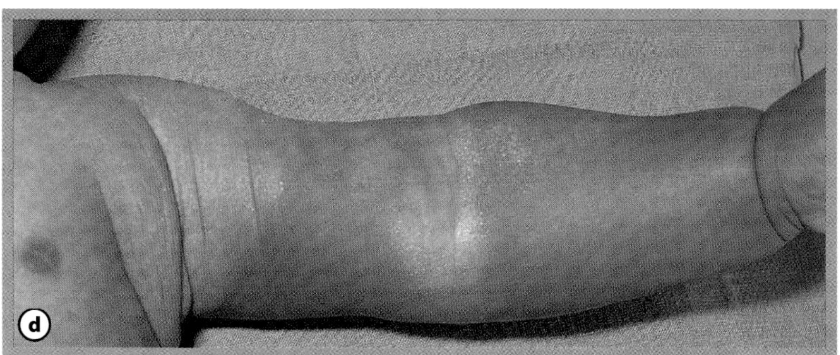

4.15a, 4.15b, 4.15c and 4.15d Infantile eczema
Infantile eczema is characterized by dryness and hyperpigmentation in this Asian baby. Follow-up slides (**4.15c** and **4.15d**) show areas of post-inflammatory hypopigmentation which is also common. The fundamental principle of treatment is the maintenance of moisture in the skin because dryness leads to a cycle of itching, excoriation and infection. Baseline treatment consists of frequent topical applications of generous quantities of emollient agents and oil and avoidance of all soaps. Short courses of steroid ointments may be necessary for inflammatory exacerbation, using the lowest potency possible, in infants usually 1% or occasionally 2.5%.

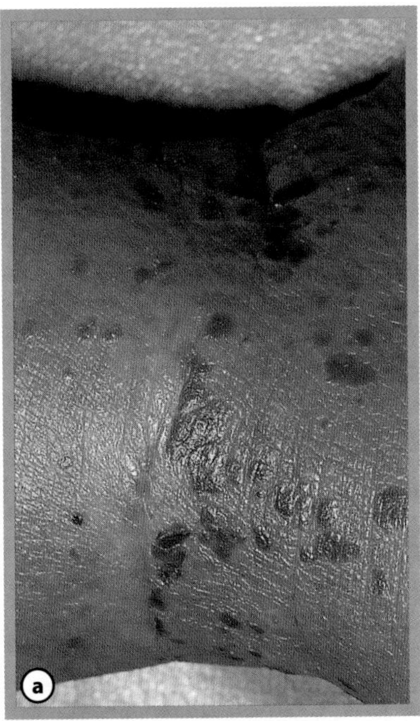

4.16a and 4.16b Eczema herpeticum

Infective exacerbation (as shown) should be treated with oral antibiotics covering streptococcus and staphylococcal strains; avoid topical antibiotics. In addition always consider the possibility of herpetic infection, as indeed was the case in this infant, which requires systemic acyclovir, usually intravenous, unless the affected area is very localized and the infant is extremely well.

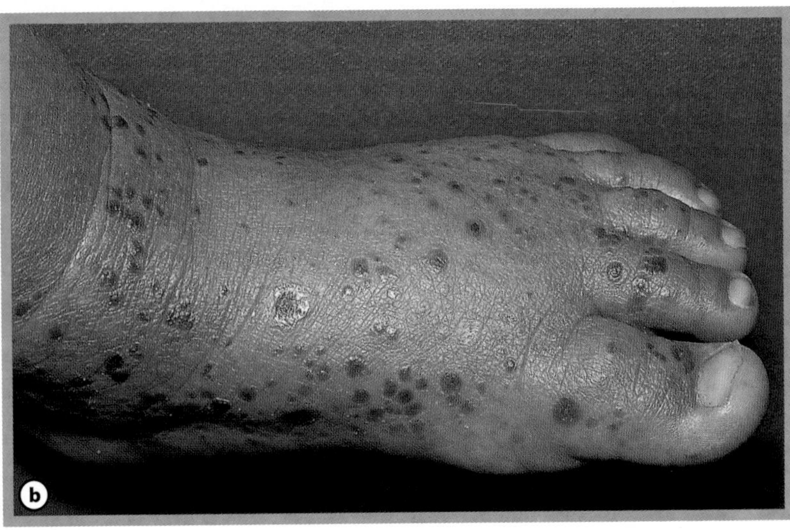

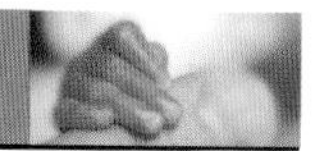

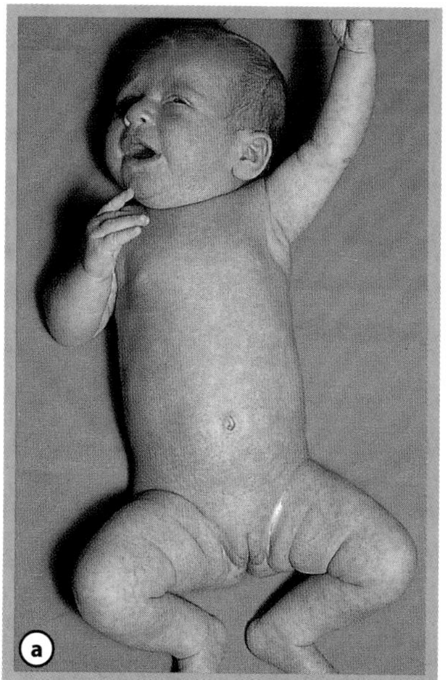

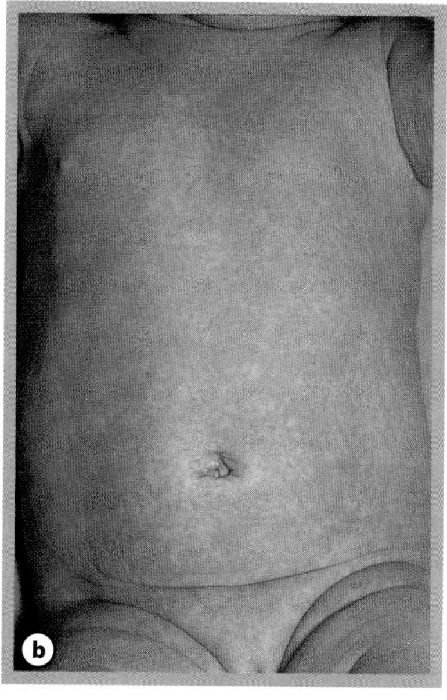

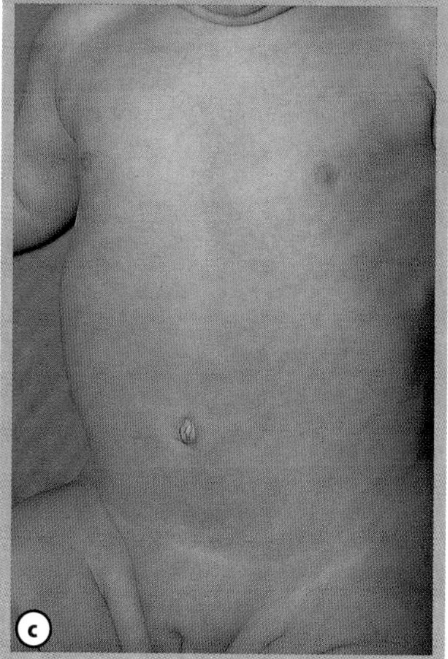

4.17a, 4.17b and 4.17c Milk allergy
This infant presented with a widespread erythematous scaly rash within the first 6 weeks of life. After 2 weeks the rash worsened (**4.17b**) and topical steroid and antifungal agents were given. No improvement occurred and in view of a tenuous history of 'milk allergy' within the extended family, the mother persuaded the doubting paediatrician to switch the infant to soya milk, with dramatic effects visible within 3 days (**4.17c**).

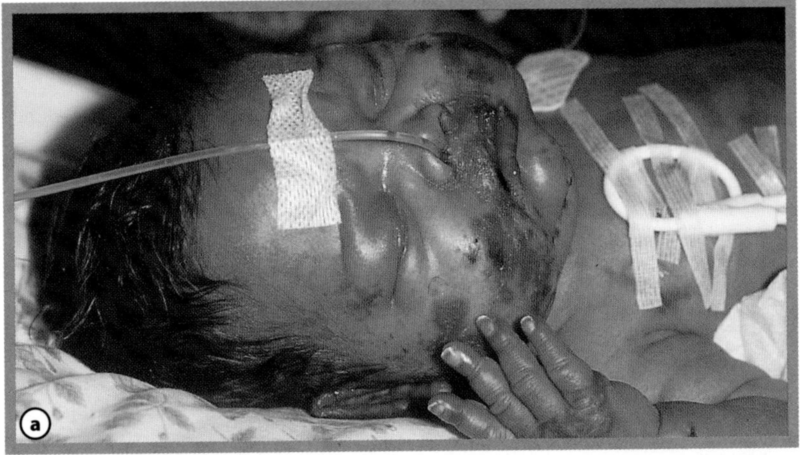

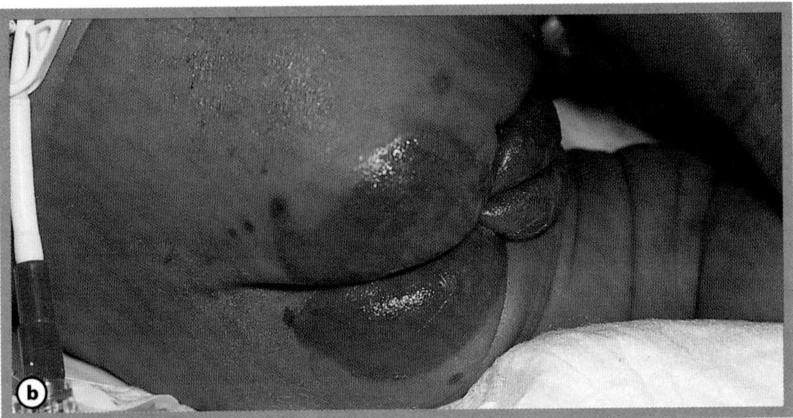

4.18a and 4.18b Acrodermatitis enteropathica
The classical features of zinc deficiency caused by this autosomal recessive condition are shown. A severe erosive mucositis is present involving the oral mucosa and perianal area. The condition is caused by an impairment of zinc absorption from the gut and associated failure to thrive is common. Alkaline phosphatase is often low because it is a zinc-dependent enzyme. Treatment is with oral zinc supplements; in the case of infants on long-term total parenteral nutrition who develop a similar clinical pattern, increased zinc supplementation of the parenteral regimen is needed.

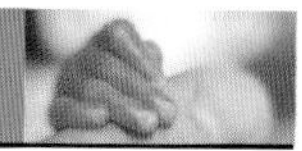

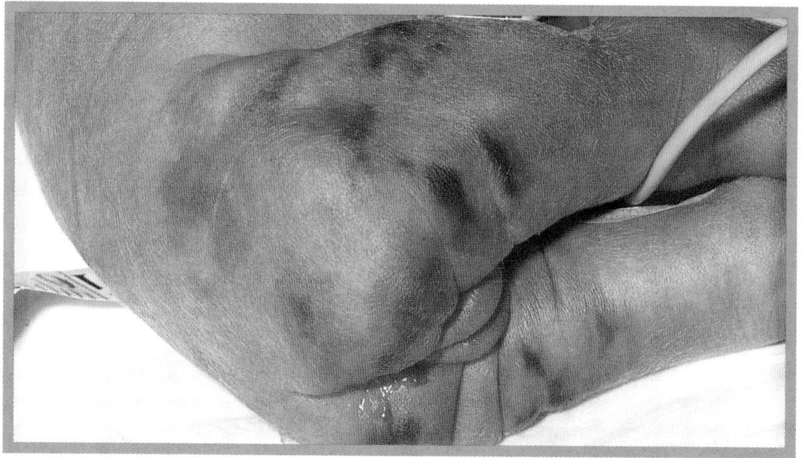

4.19 Congenital Gram-negative sepsis
This infant presented with collapse, shock and a fulminant purpuric rash within the first few hours of life. Gram-negative septicaemia was found to be the cause of the illness, which in neonates may run a course very similar to meningococcal sepsis with profound shock, capillary leak syndrome and disseminated intra-vascular coagulation. Mortality from this condition is high.

4.20 Congenital cytomegalovirus
This infant presented with purpura associated with thrombocytopaenia and hepatosplenomegaly caused by congenital cytomegalovirus. Asymptomatic cytomegalovirus infection in the mother is common and fewer than 10% of infants are affected, the majority of which have no clinical adverse effects. However, some infants are severely affected with microcephaly, periventricular calcification and disseminated features, as is this infant.

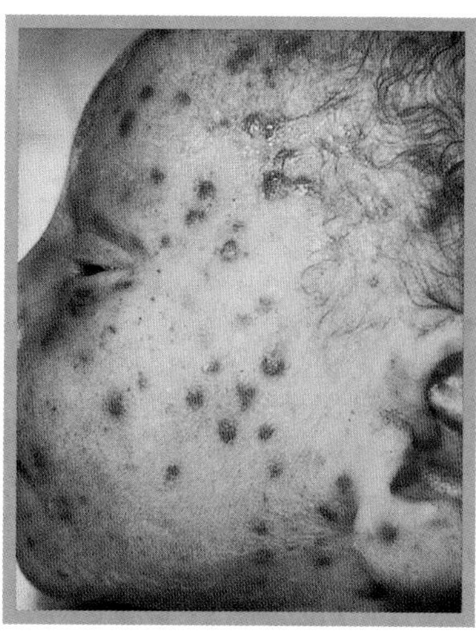

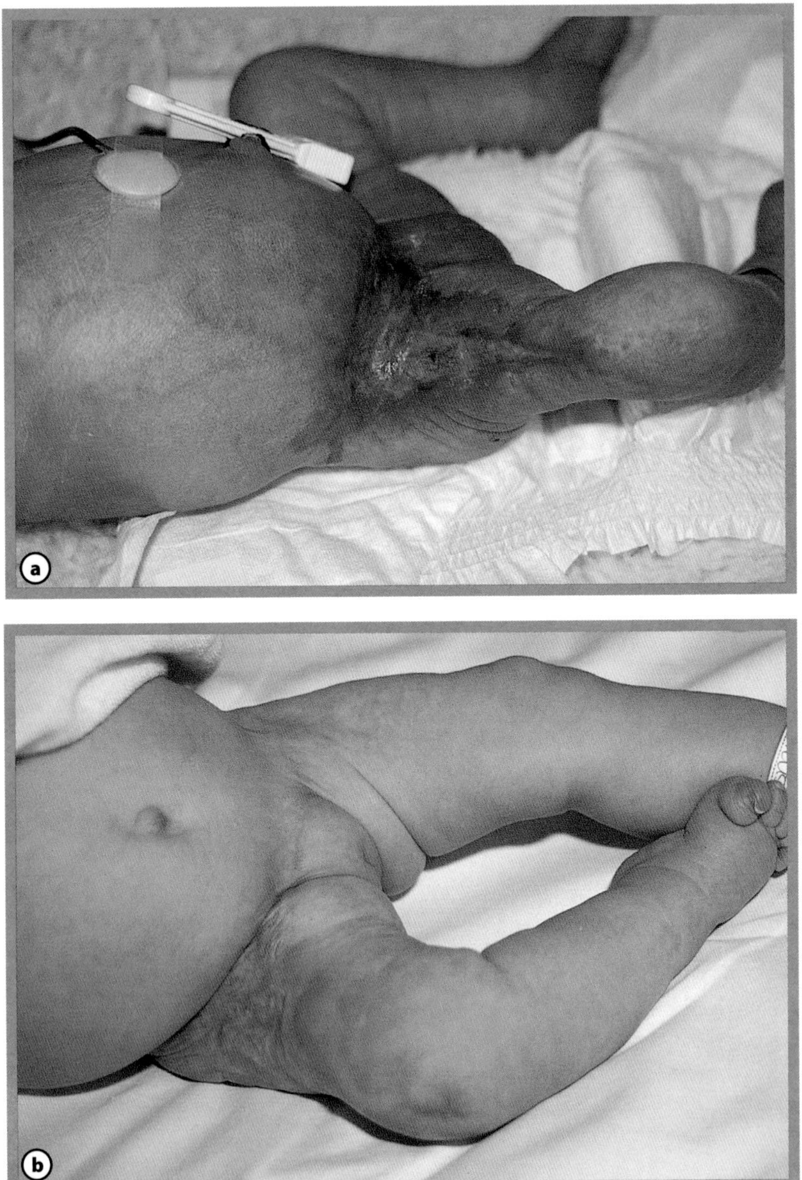

a

b

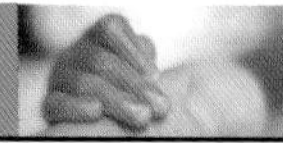

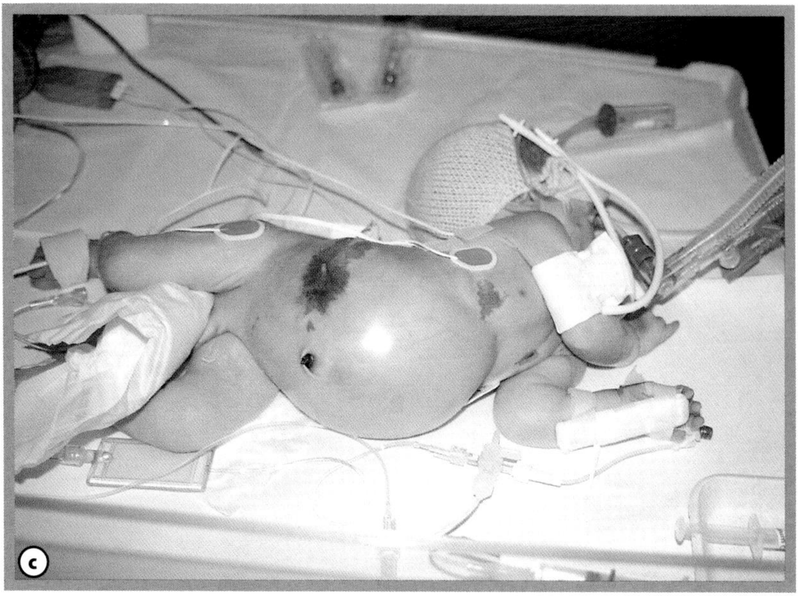

4.21a, 4.21b and 4.21c Congenital varicella

Although this is rare, there is a well-defined syndrome of congenital varicella after exposure of a mother to varicella for the first time during pregnancy, usually within the first 20 weeks. One of the well documented features of this condition, extensive cutaneous eruption is shown in **4.21a**. The follow-up slide (**4.21b**) shows healing with scar formation. Other features of congenital varicella include severe neuro disability, limb defects and eye abnormalities. Disseminated varicella may occur as shown in **4.21c** with hepatosplenomegaly and respiratory failure.

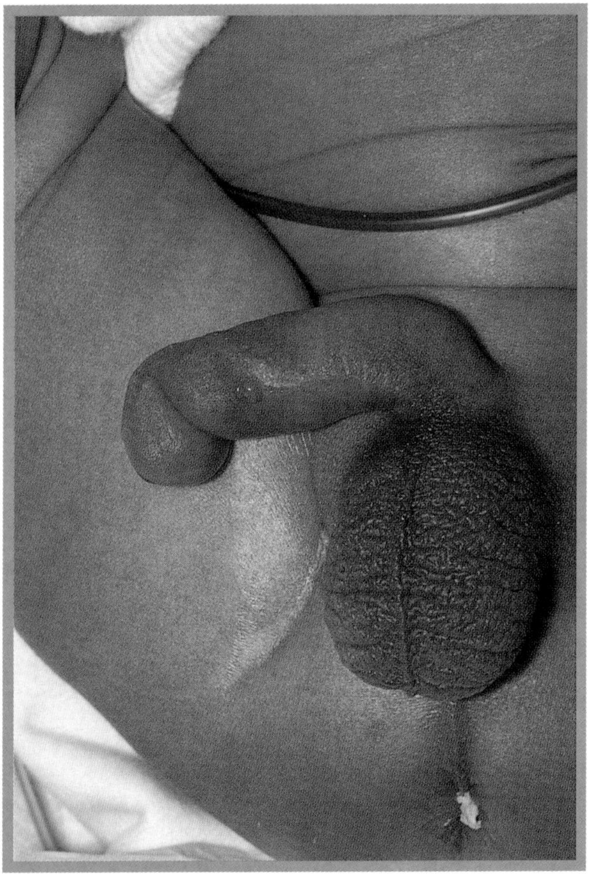

4.22 Neonatal herpes

An isolated vesicle on the penis is shown and is part of neonatal herpetic illness acquired *intra-partum*. The infection may be localized to the skin as in this case, may result in meningoencephalitis or in severe cases result in a systemic illness with thrombocytopaenia, disseminated intra-vascular coagulation and hepatosplenomegaly. Treatment is with intravenous acyclovir.

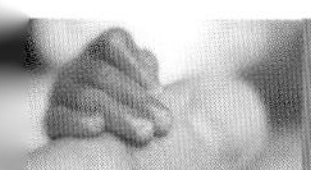

5 Head and neck

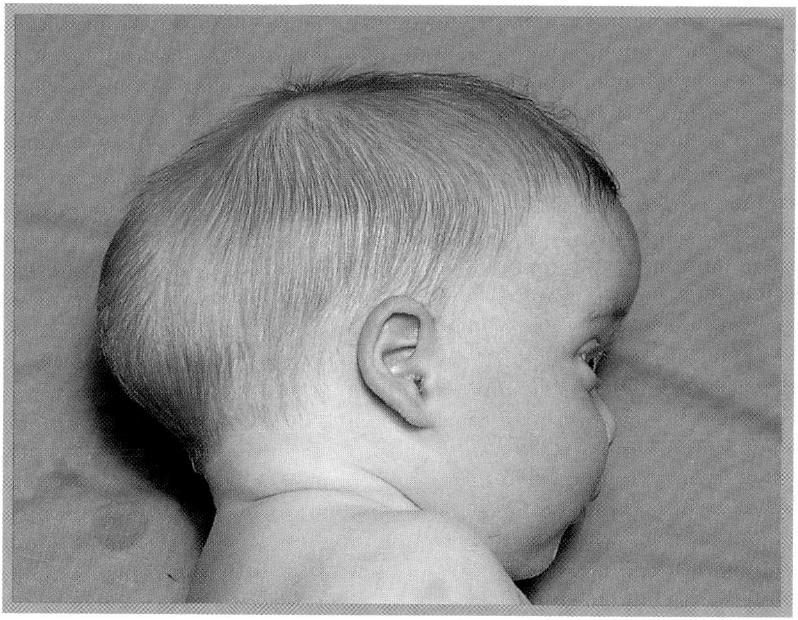

5.1 Scaphocephaly
This is the most common form of craniosynostosis, involving premature closure of the sagittal suture. The main findings are a prominent occiput and a broad forehead and either a small or absent anterior fontanelle. The main problem is cosmetic, as raised intra-cranial pressure is not usually a feature.

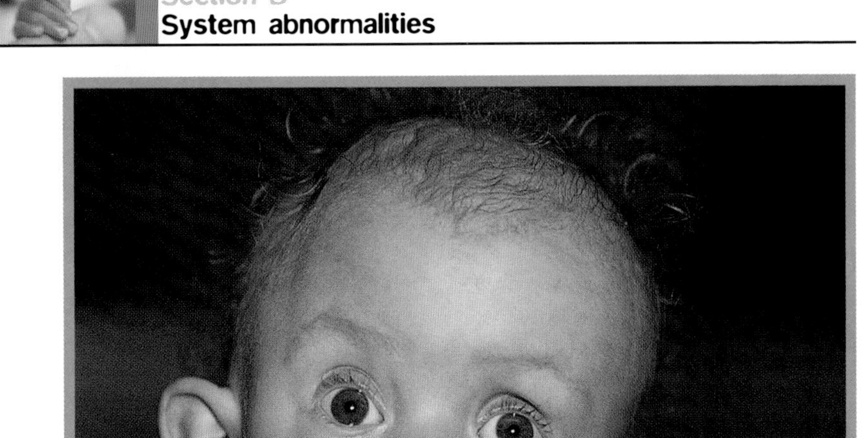

5.2a, 5.2b and 5.2c Unicoronal craniosynostosis
Closure of the coronal suture, sphenofrontal suture or both leads to unilateral flattening of the forehead, elevation of the ipsilateral orbit and eyebrow as well as a prominent ear on the corresponding side. In the severe form, which is rare, surgery produces good results. The X-ray (**5.2b**) and the reconstructed three-dimensional computerized tomography scan (**5.2c**) clearly shows the fused right coronal suture.

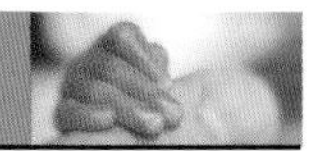

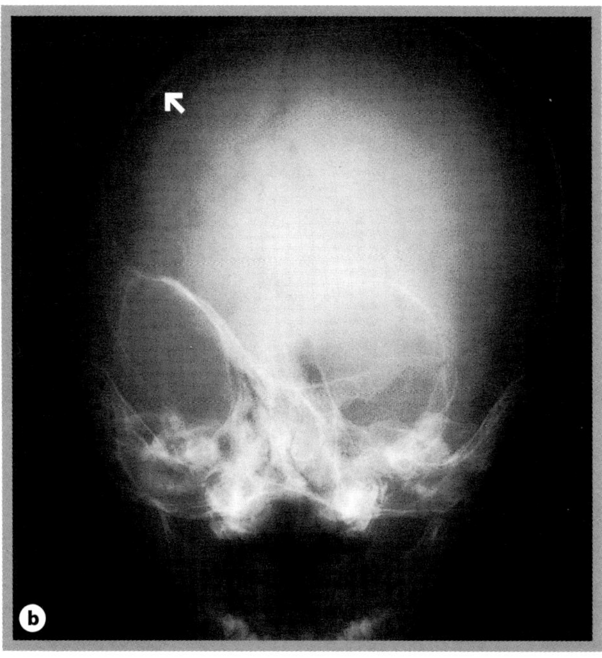

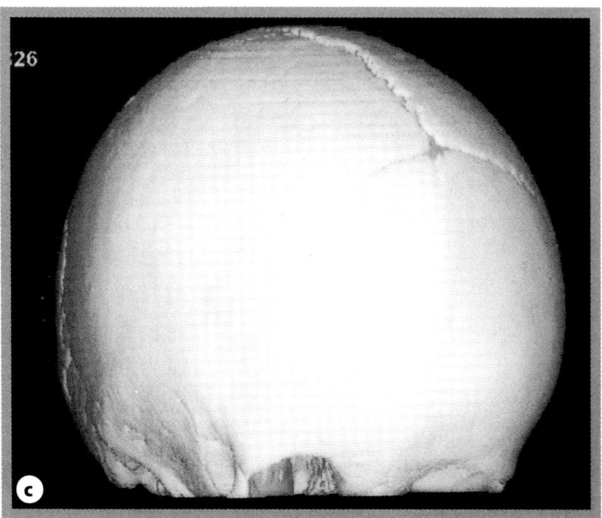
26

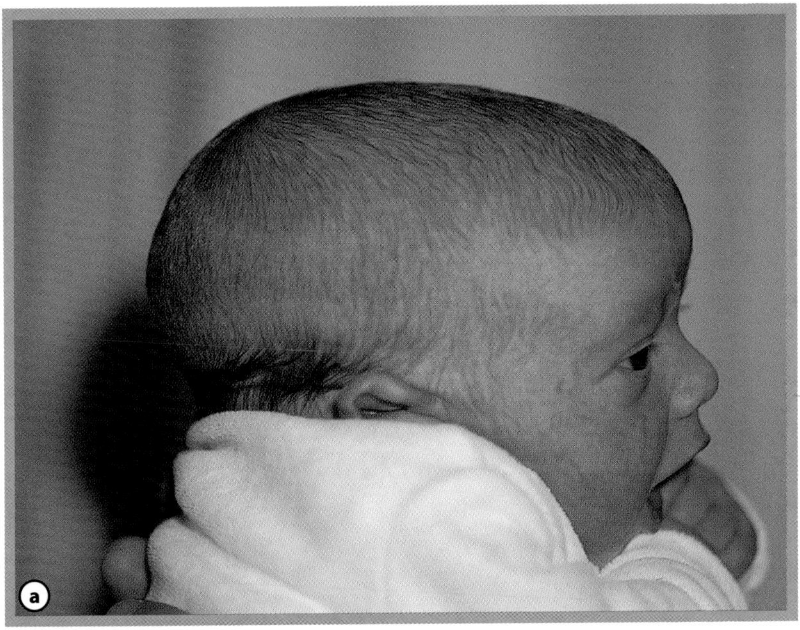

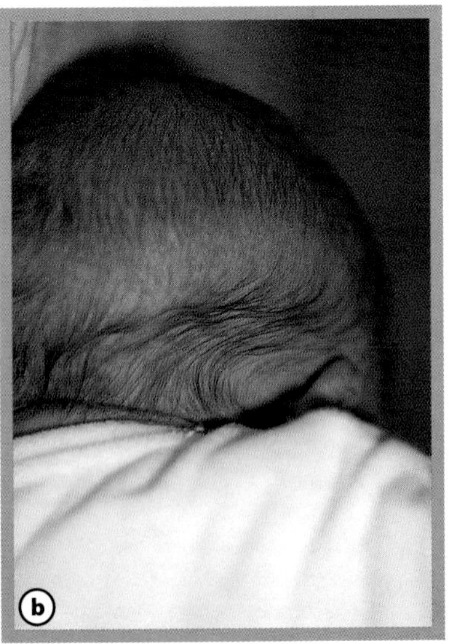

5.3a, 5.3b, 5.3c and 5.3d Occipital plagiocephaly
Intra-uterine moulding caused this infant's skull shape. The skull radiograph (**5.3c**) confirms the shape of the head and the presence of open sutures excluding craniosynostosis. A gradual return to a normal head shape will occur over subsequent months. This form of plagiocephaly is more commonly seen because of positioning either *in utero* or in infancy in an immobile child. The likely position that the infant maintained *in utero* is shown (**5.3d**).

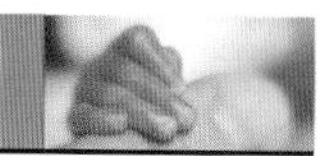

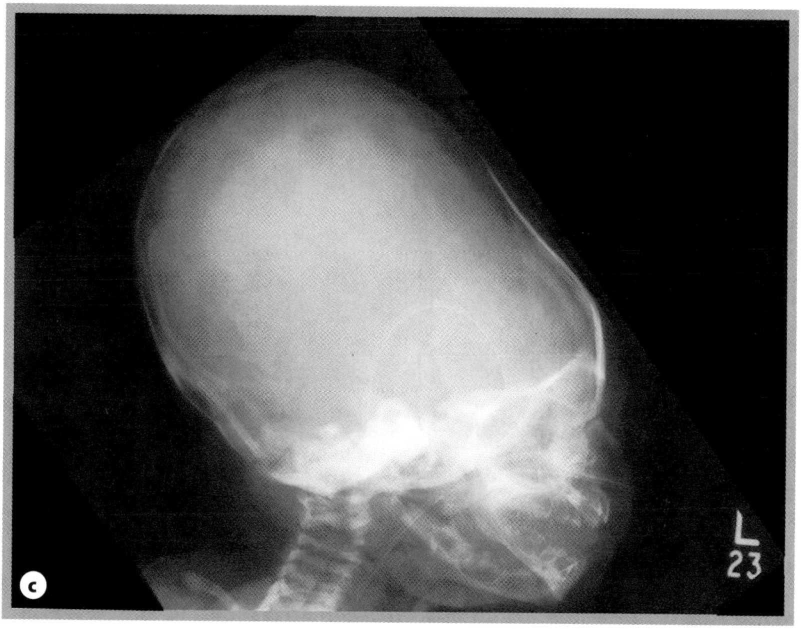

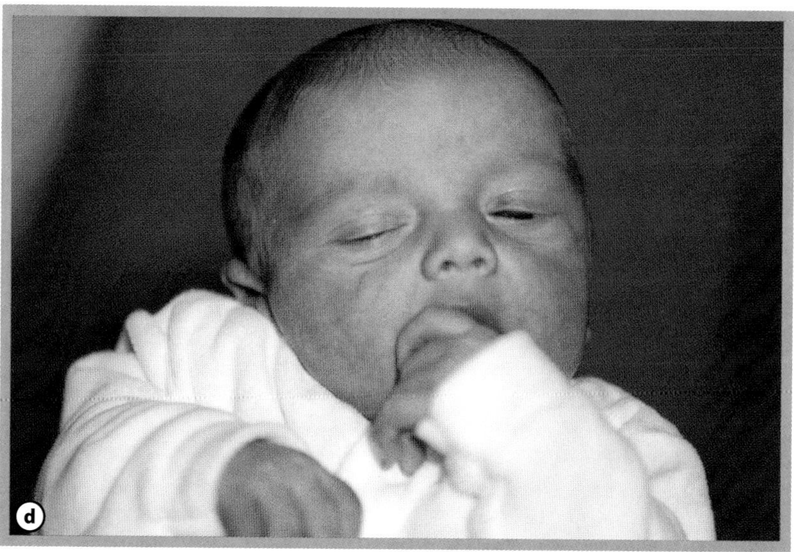
d

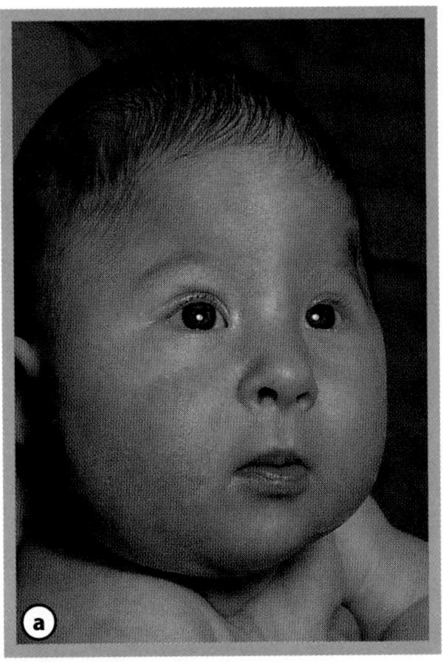

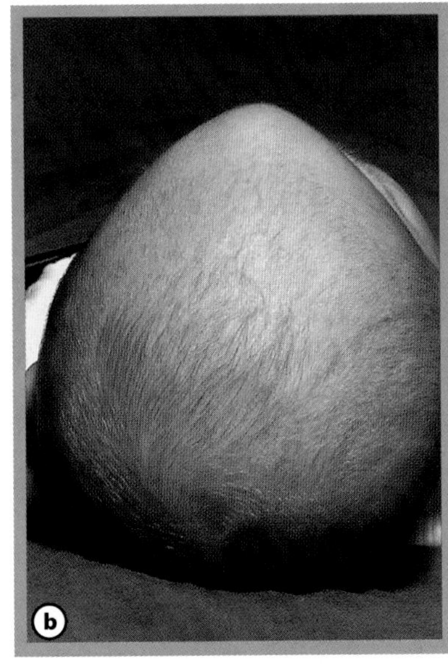

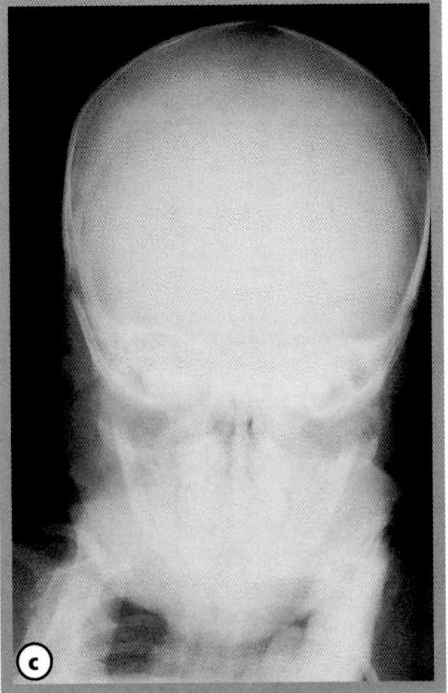

5.4a, 5.4b and 5.4c Trigonocephaly

This abnormality is rare and is often caused by ridging or fusion of the metopic suture. The associated facial feature is orbital hypertelorism. In addition, there is a risk of associated developmental abnormalities of the forebrain. The skull X-ray shows the fused metopic suture.

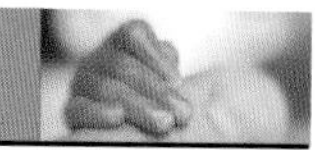

5.5 Brachycephaly

This can be a normal variant, as in the radiograph shown, or occur as a result of closure of both coronal sutures, leading to antero-posterior shortening of the skull. The facial appearance is characteristic with prominent, wide-set eyes; the face itself appears flat and broad. There is a strong association with defects such as cleft palate, syndactyly and polydactyly as well as cerebral abnormalities. Patients with Down syndrome commonly have brachycephaly without synostosis.

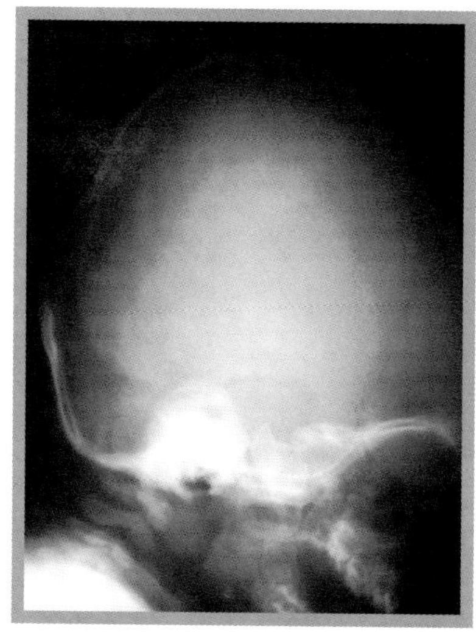

5.6 Angular dermoid cyst

An angular dermoid cyst is usually situated at the outer angle of the eyebrow area. This cyst was unusually placed at the inner angle of the eye. A computerized tomography scan confirmed this cyst to have an intra-cranial extension.

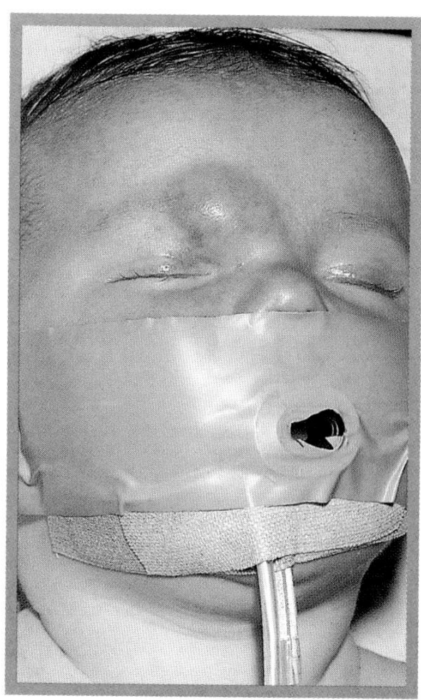

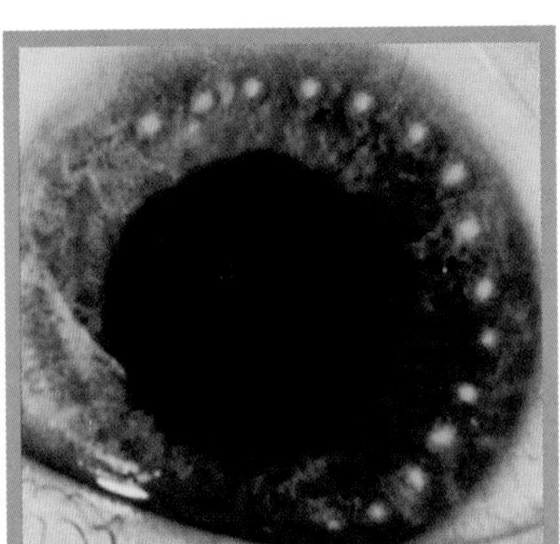

5.7 Brushfield spots

Brushfield spots occur in about 50% of patients with Down syndrome. They occur as a result of focal areas of iris stromal hyperplasia surrounded by relative hypoplasia.

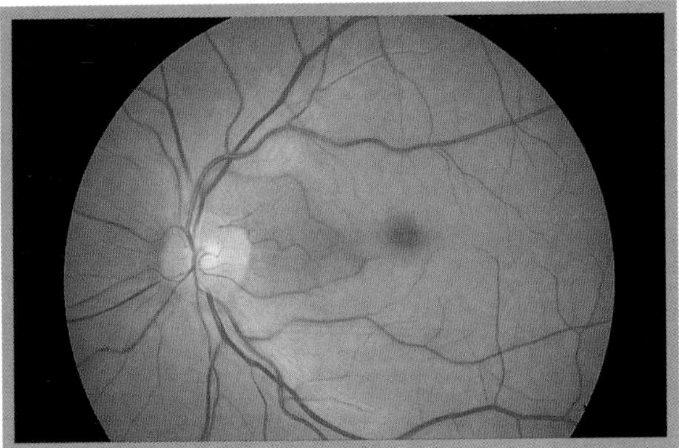

5.8 Cherry red spot

This typical appearance is caused by either loss of transparency of the extrafoveal retina due to extracellular or intra-cellular oedema or deposition of abnormal metabolic by-products in the retinal ganglion cells. As the ganglion cells are only one layer thick or even absent in the macular area, it is here that the 'red spot' is visible. Examples of conditions where a red spot is seen are Niemann–Pick or Tay–Sachs disease (as in this infant).

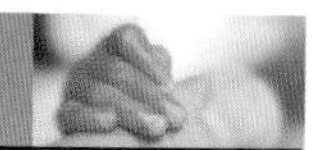

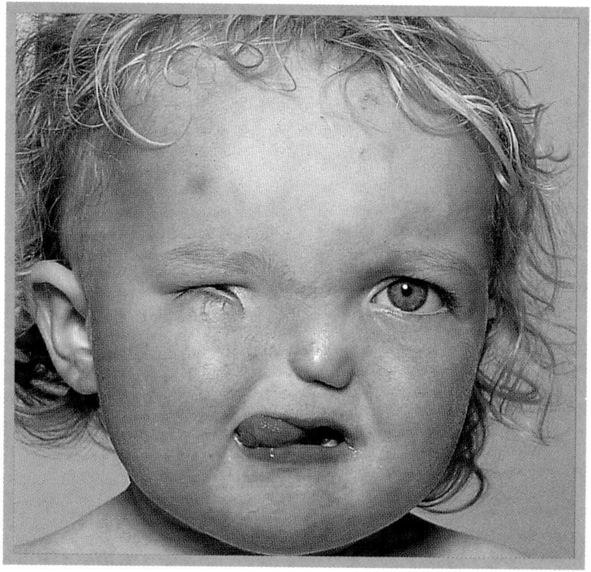

5.9 Anophthalmos
This patient had complete absence of the right globe. This condition may occur sporadically but may also be part of a chromosomal disorder such as trisomy 13. In rare cases it may be inherited as an autosomal dominant trait.

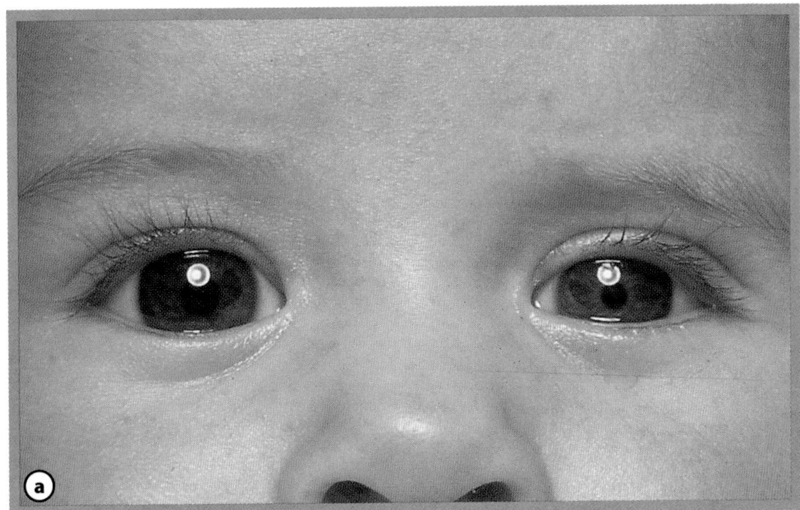

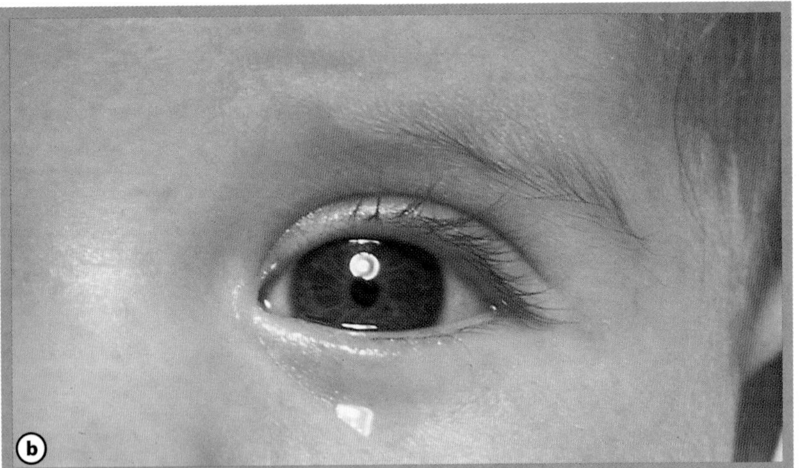

5.10a and 5.10b Horner syndrome
Features shown are ptosis, miosis and anhidrosis. It may be congenital or secondary to stretching of the sympathetic cervical fibres during traumatic delivery. Recovery depends on whether nerve stretching or transection occurred.

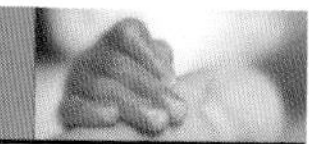

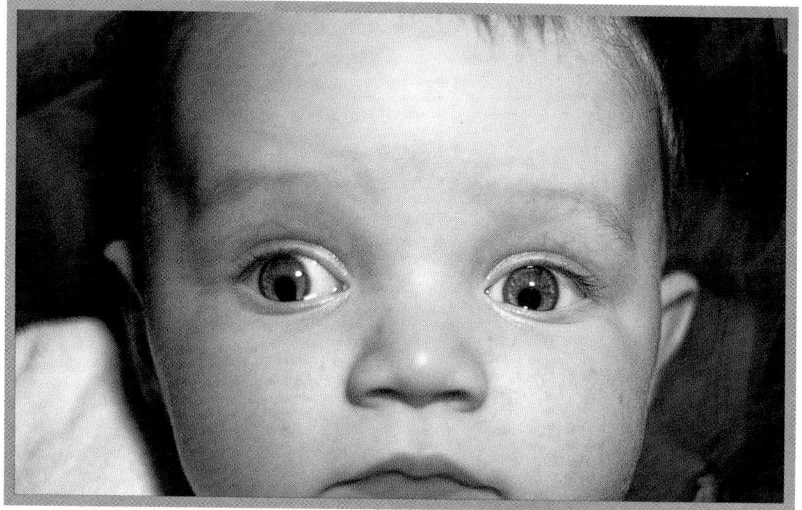

5.11 Coloboma
Defects in the iris may occur in isolation or in association with a wide range of chromosomal abnormalities (e.g. trisomy 13) or other sequences (e.g. CHARGE). The lesion may be limited to the iris, usually the inferior part at 6 o'clock as shown, and have little effect on vision. However, it may reflect an underlying defect extending to the fundus and optic nerve tract in which case vision may be severely impaired.

5.12 Congenital cataract
Cataracts may be difficult to diagnose in the early neonatal period because most infants spend a great deal of time asleep; in addition their pupils are usually small. It is important in the examination of the newborn specifically to check for the red reflex. This infant has a unilateral cataract secondary to congenital rubella.

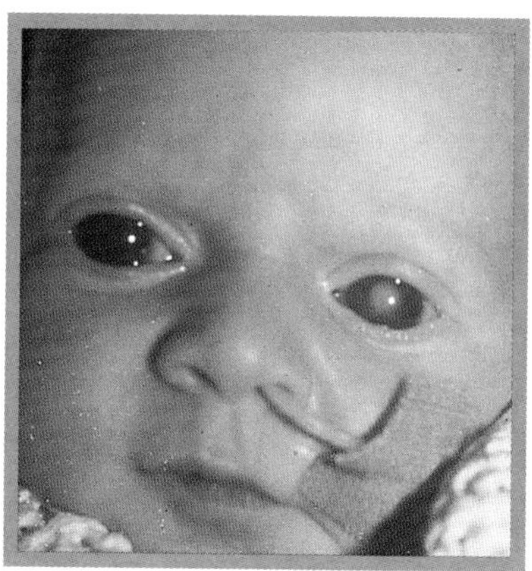

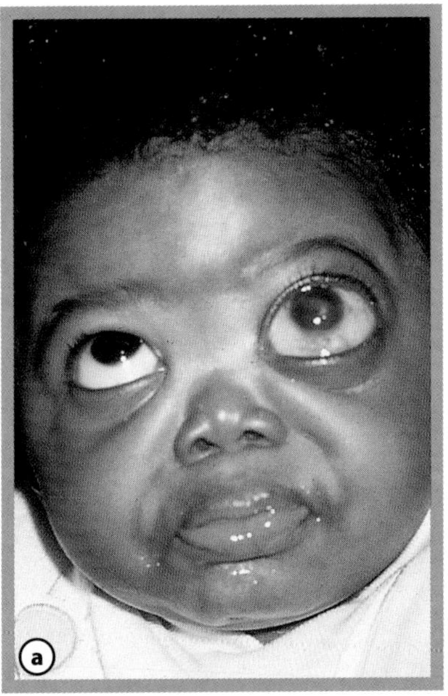

5.13a and 5.13b Congenital glaucoma

These infants show marked proptosis and enlargement of the eye, 'buphthalmos', in association with congenital glaucoma. The intra-ocular pressure is raised and blindness may result from effects on the optic nerve unless the pressure can be controlled. Congenital glaucoma is associated with numerous conditions, for example, Sturge–Weber syndrome, aniridia and intra-ocular tumours.

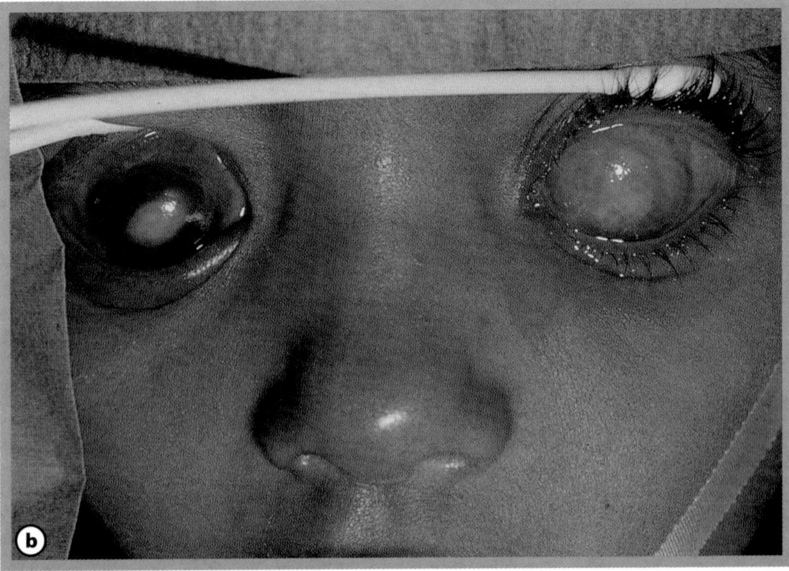

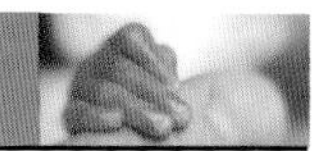

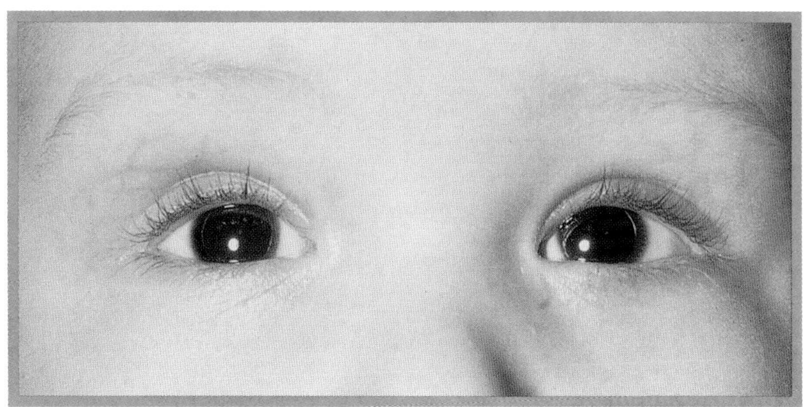

5.14 Aniridia

Congenital absence of the iris, which may be due to deletion of the p13 region of chromosome 11, is illustrated. Inheritance may be either autosomal dominant or sporadic. The sporadic form is associated with an increased risk of developing Wilms' tumour.

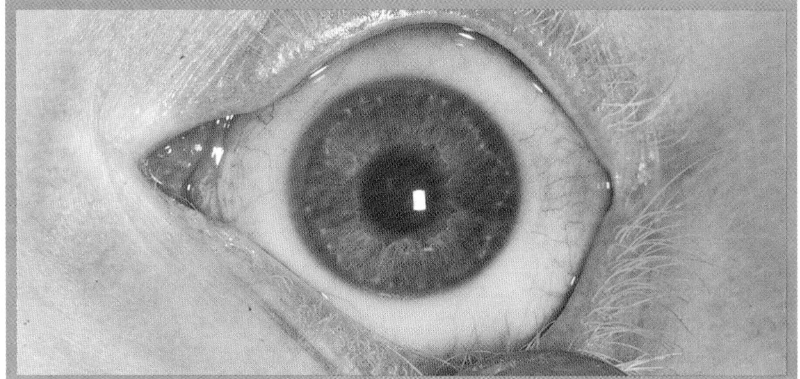

5.15 Ocular albinism

This infant shows the typical features of albinism: translucency of the iris and a very blond fundus due to lack of pigment in the epithelium. Clinically, these infants show nystagmus and poor visual responses which improve in later childhood.

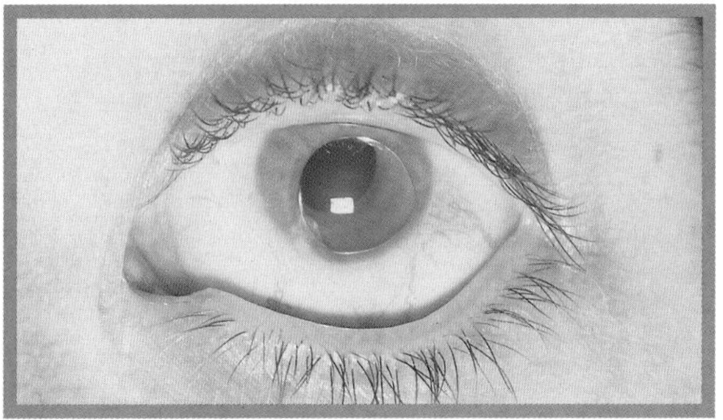

5.16 Dislocation of the lens
This is often found in patients with homocystinuria or with Marfan syndrome. Subluxation of the lens in Marfan syndrome occurs more commonly in the superior direction whereas in homocystinuria it occurs more commonly in the inferior direction. This infant has downward subluxation.

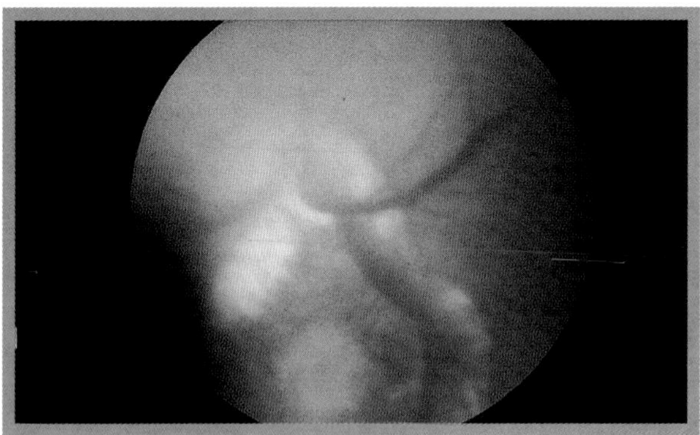

5.17 Congenital toxoplasmosis
This slide shows the fundus of an infant with congenital toxoplasmosis and demonstrates the typical findings of choroidoretinitis. All infants born to mothers who may have acquired toxoplasmosis during pregnancy must have formal fundoscopy in the neonatal period because combined chemotherapy may prove sight-saving in affected neonates.

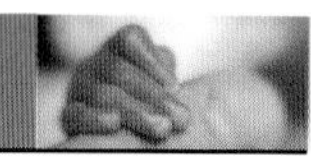

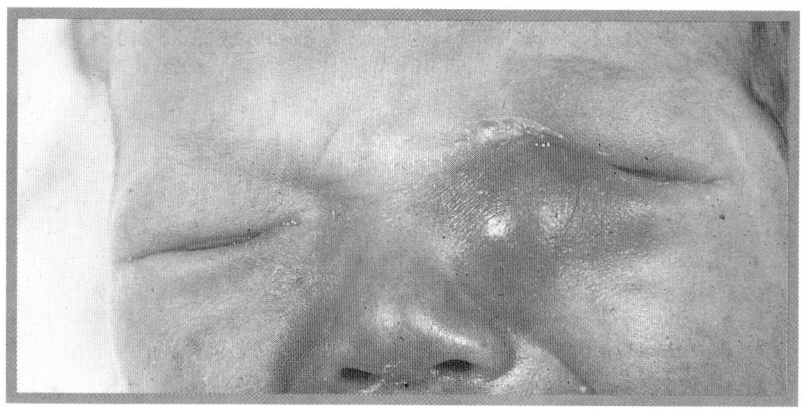

5.18 Dacrocystitis
This infant shows redness and swelling of the nasolacrimal duct with secondary conjunctivitis. Systemic antibiotics are required and surgery may be necessary to relieve the obstruction of the nasolacrimal duct.

5.19 Hemifacial microsomia
In this condition there is an underdevelopment of the mandible, gross hypoplasia or aplasia of the pinna of the ear with a blind or absent external auditory meatus. Flattening of the face on the affected side is due to aplasia of the mandibular ramus and condyle as well as a deficiency in the maxillary and malar bones. The muscles of facial expression and mastication may also be hypoplastic. No obvious pattern of inheritance is identified.

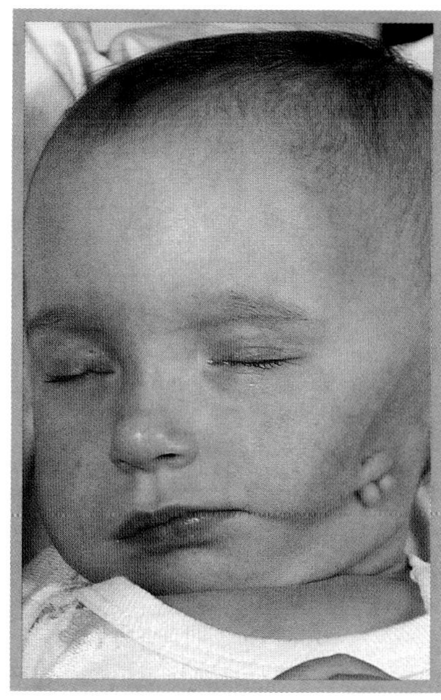

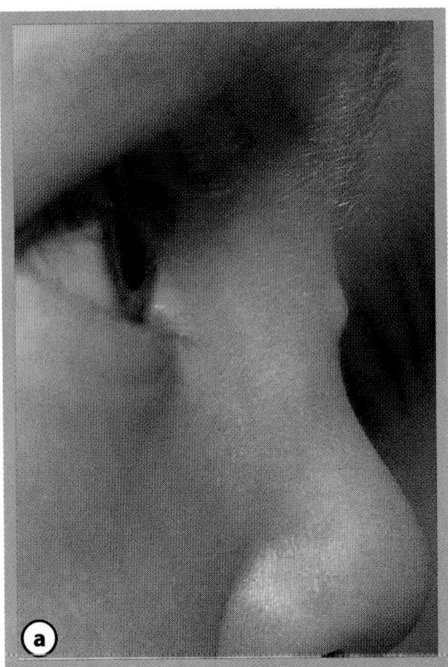

5.20a and 5.20b Dermoid cyst
These cysts usually occur on the face or scalp and represent internalized epithelial cells and may contain cartilage or bone.

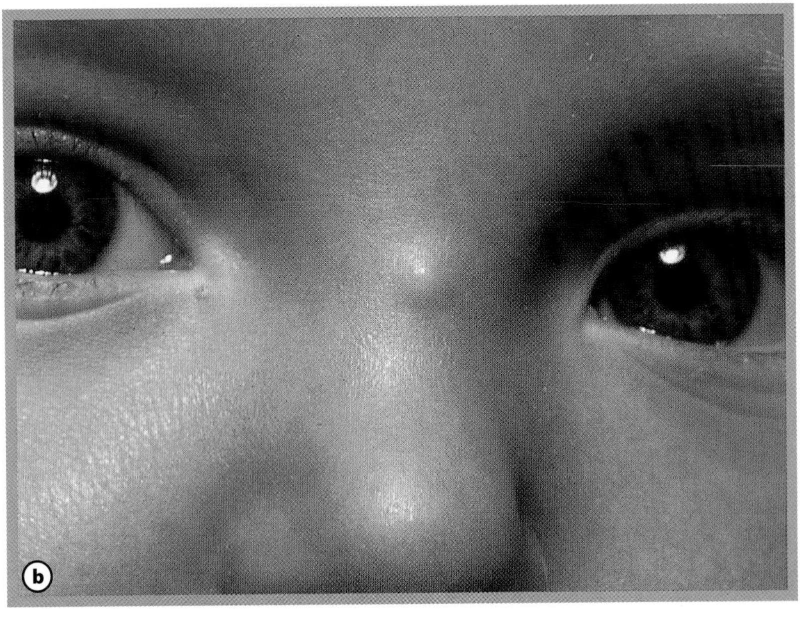

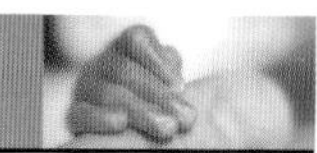

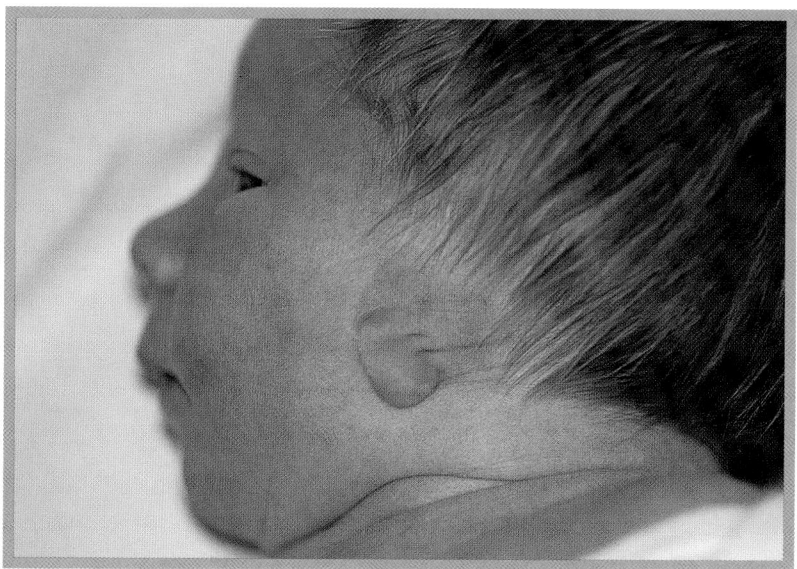

5.21 Congenital absence of ear

This infant has atresis of the auricle and external auditory canal. Magnetic resonance imaging and audiological testing are needed to establish whether the middle ear structures are present and thus offering a prognosis for hearing on the affected side. It may occur as an isolated finding or in association with a variety of conditions, for example, Treacher Collins syndrome.

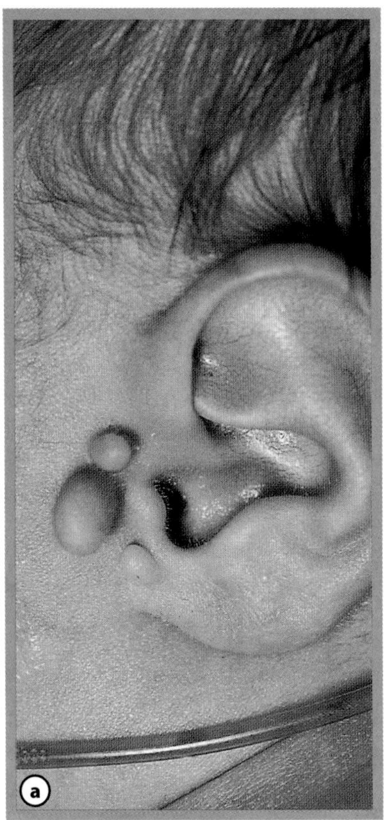

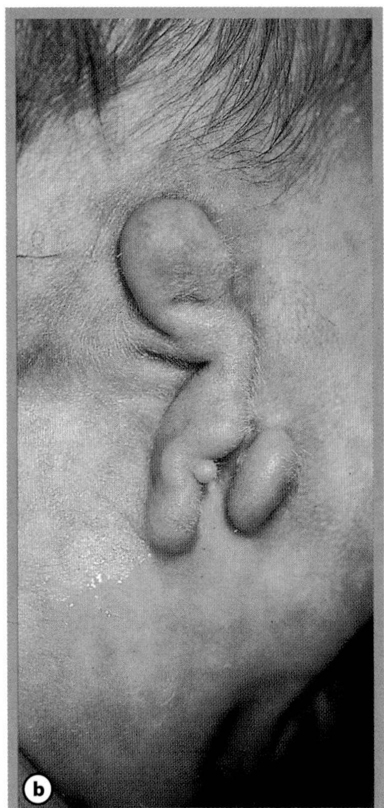

5.22a and 5.22b Goldenhar syndrome
In this syndrome pre-auricular skin tags are associated with facial hypoplasia and cervical vertebral defects.

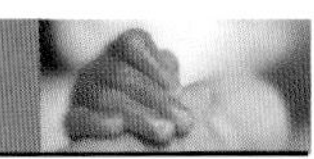

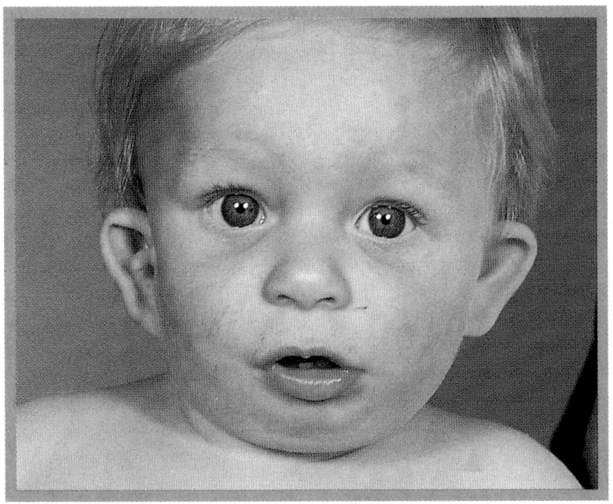

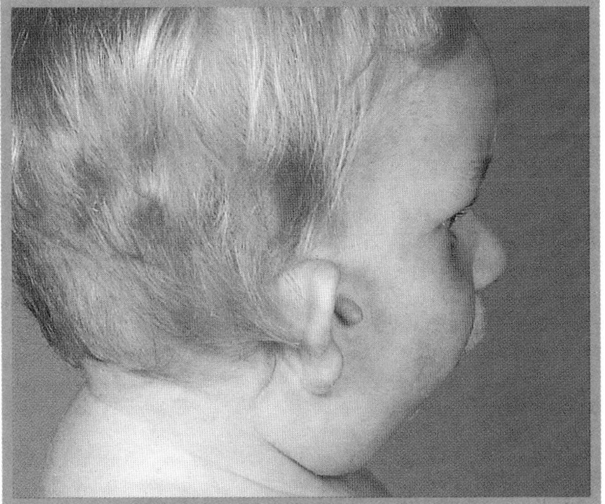

5.23a and 5.23b Treacher Collins syndrome
In this autosomal dominant condition, there are abnormalities of the external ear and auditory canal in association with a classical facies caused by mandibular and mid-facial hypoplasia.

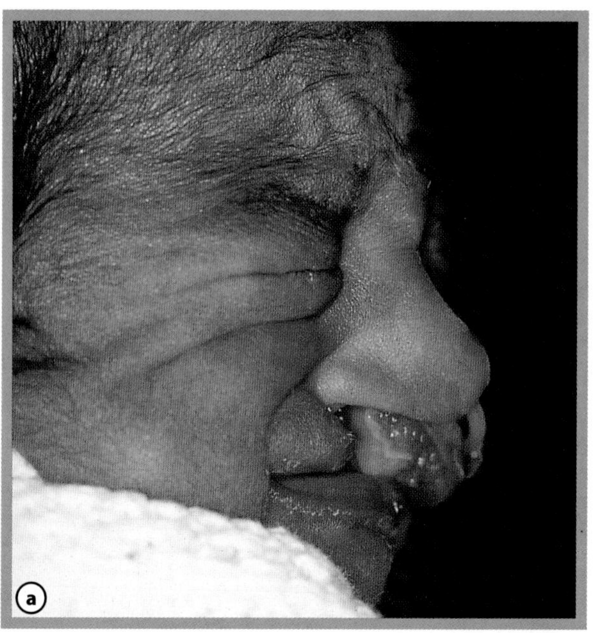

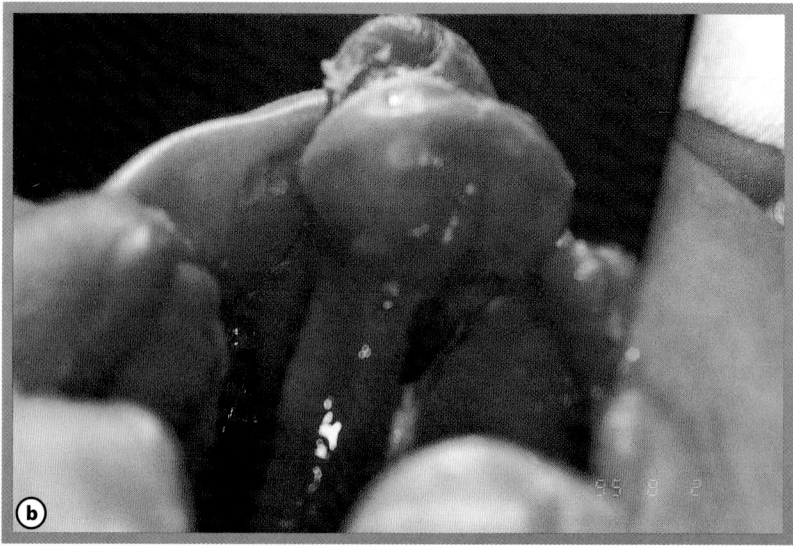

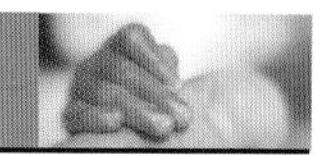

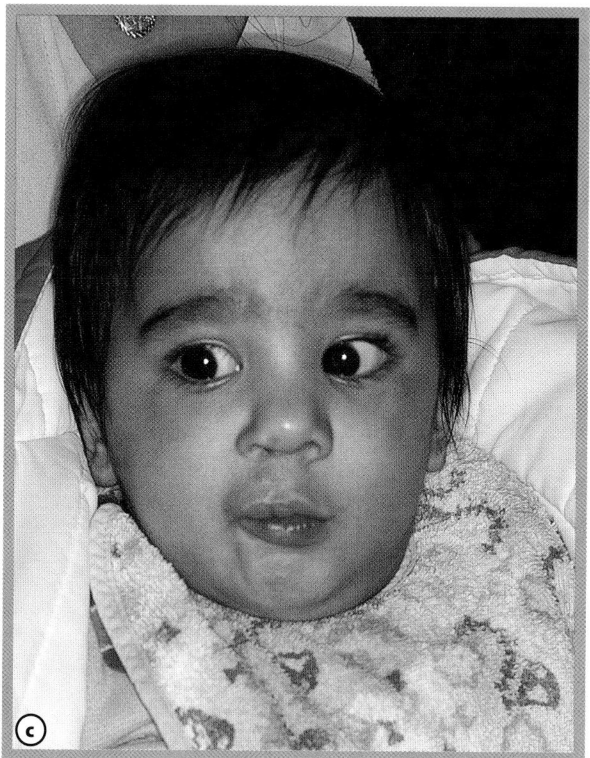

5.24a, 5.24b and 5.24c Cleft lip
A cleft lip may be bilateral and associated with a cleft palate (as shown) or cleft nares. The image in **5.24b** has been taken with a mirror within the oral cavity. Inheritance is polygenic and antenatal diagnosis and surgical correction may be undertaken. Early correction within the first week is now advocated. A photograph 2 years later (**5.24c**) shows the excellent long-term result of plastic surgery for correction of a cleft lip.

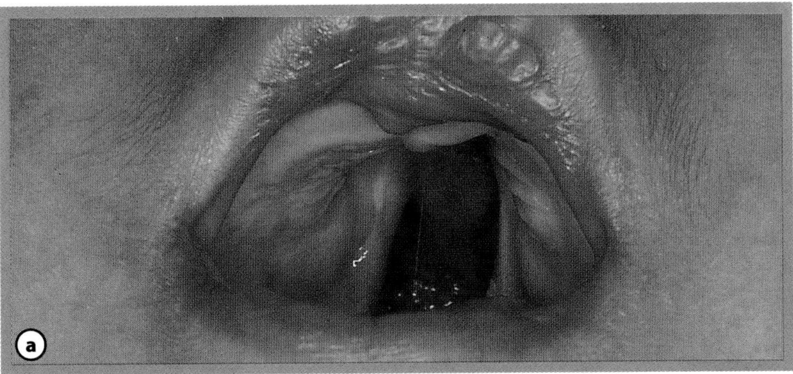

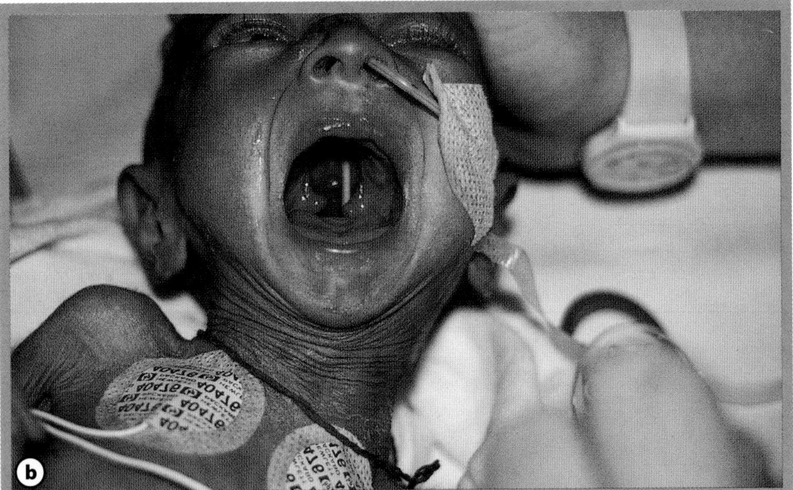

5.25a and 5.25b Cleft palate
A cleft palate may occur in isolation or in association with cleft lip or syndromes, for example, Pierre Robin sequence. The cleft may involve only the soft palate or extend through the hard palate and into the incisive foramen as shown in these two patients. The main early complication is poor feeding and severe failure to thrive may follow as shown in **5.25b**. Treatment is multidisciplinary including craniofacial and maxillofacial surgeons, speech therapists and orthodontists. Long-term speech and hearing problems may occur despite corrective surgery, as may maxillofacial underdevelopment.

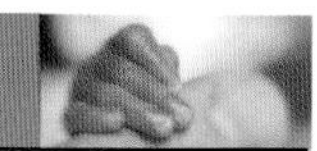

5.26a and 5.26b Pierre Robin sequence

The essential defect of Pierre Robin sequence is poor development of the mandible, resulting in retrognathia and micrognathia in association with a cleft palate. The tongue tends to fall backwards, glossoptosis, causing obstruction to the upper airway and respiratory failure. Nasopharyngeal airways are sometimes required as shown or in severe cases tracheostomy (*see* **5.28**). The tongue can be held forwards by a suture allowing time for the mandible to develop.

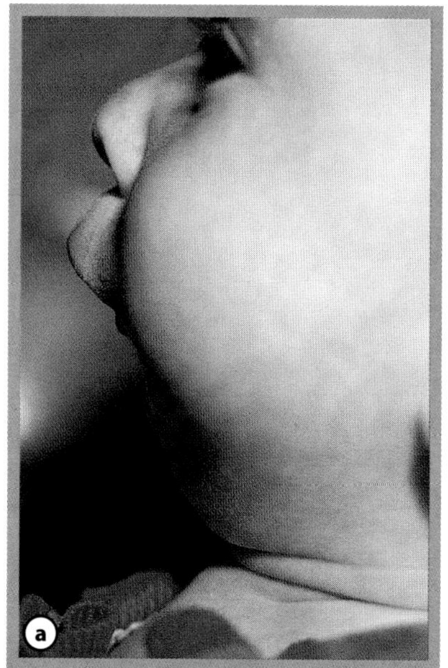

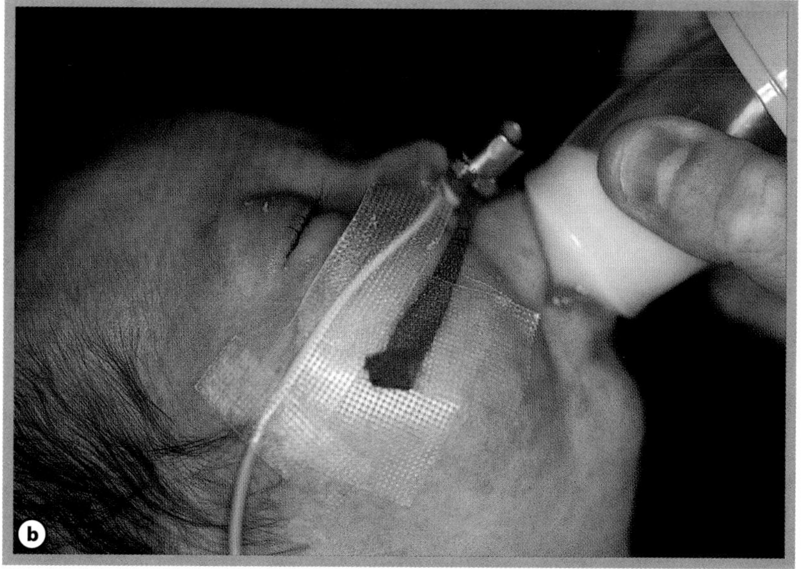

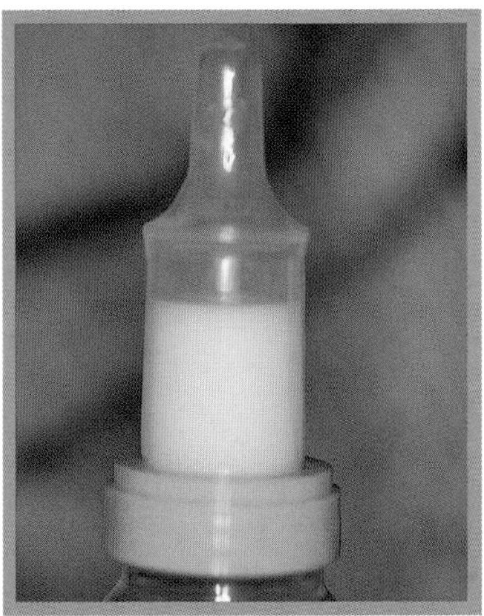

5.27 Haberman teat
A Haberman teat is shown which is a useful feeding adjunct for infants with cleft palate.

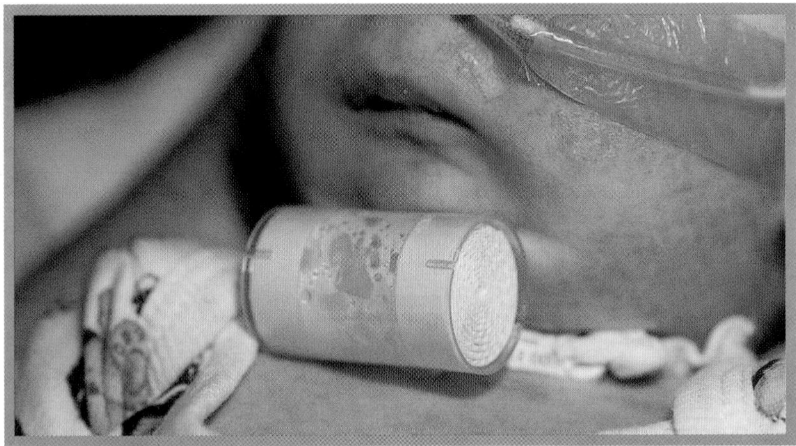

5.28 Tracheostomy
Tracheostomy was unavoidable in this infant who was diagnosed with Pierre Robin sequence antenatally. Immediately after birth endotracheal canulation was impossible because of severe upper airway obstruction. Another cause requiring a tracheostomy in neonates is repeated endotracheal intubation causing subglottal stenosis.

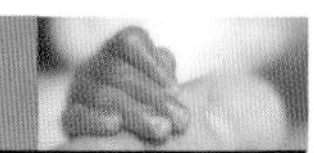

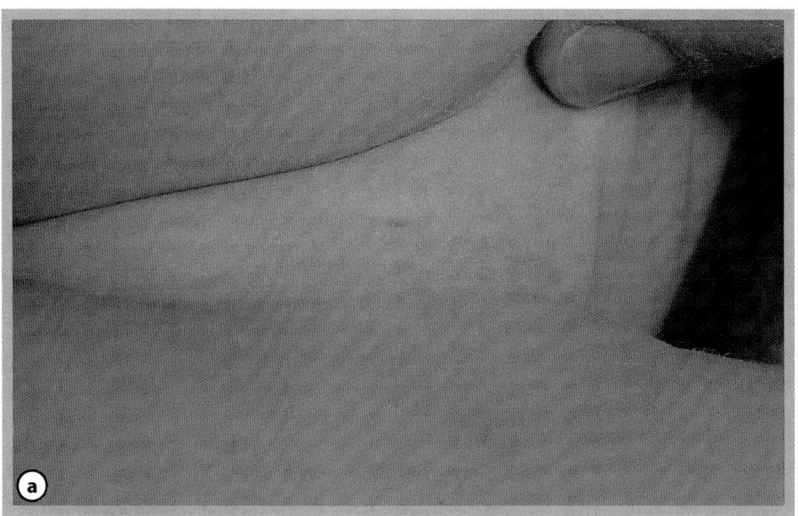

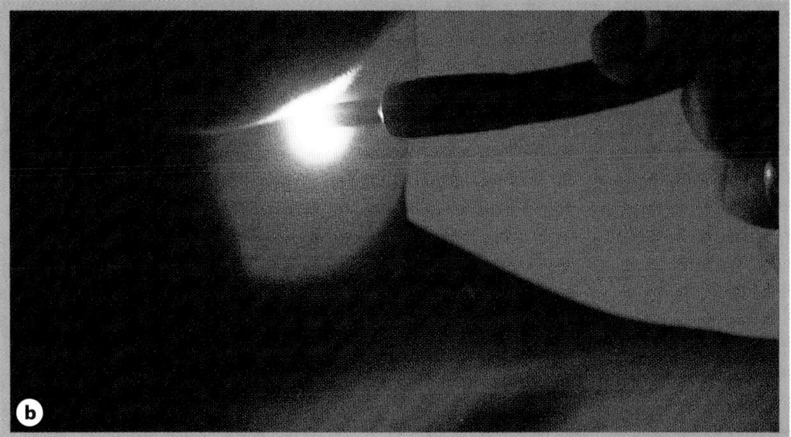

5.29a and 5.29b Branchial sinus or cyst
A branchial sinus is shown that arose from a failure of complete fusion of the branchial arches during embryonic development. Excision is required because of risk of subsequent infection including tuberculosis. A cyst may also arise by the same mechanism as shown in **5.29b** that transilluminates, differentiating it from an enlarged lymph node.

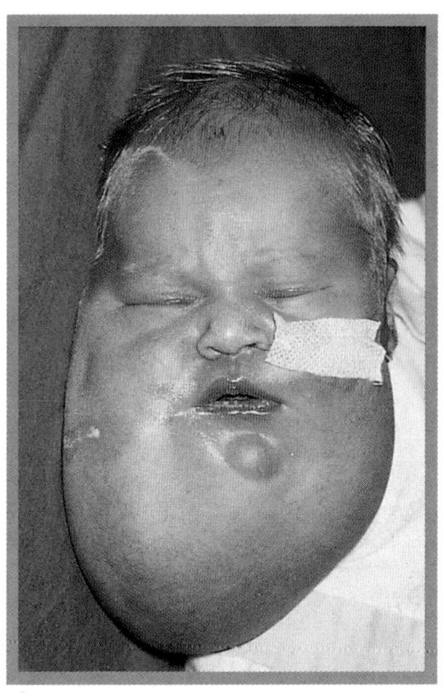

5.30 Cystic hygroma
This lymphangiomatous lesion presents as a very large, fluctuant, transilluminant swelling usually involving the head and neck, although they can be present elsewhere. It has a characteristic soft consistency and it is usually difficult to define its borders. Compression of local structures may occur, for example, the trachea causing respiratory distress. Complete surgical resection may be very difficult and often requires numerous procedures, with a risk of recurrence.

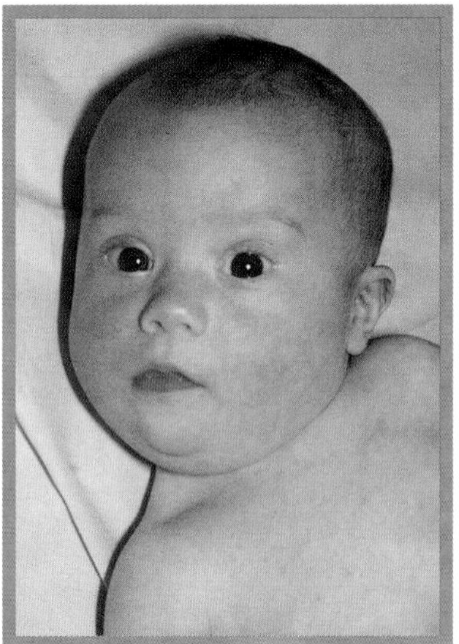

5.31 Sternomastoid tumour
The so-called sternomastoid tumour is merely a localized contraction of the sternomastoid muscle more commonly on the right, resulting in a torticollis to the left as shown. Where a bulky mass can be felt, an ultrasound is helpful to exclude a rare case of a rhabdomyosarcoma. Treatment is by physiotherapy and most cases resolve.

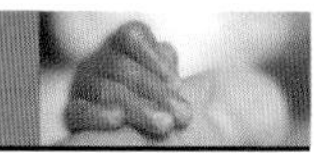

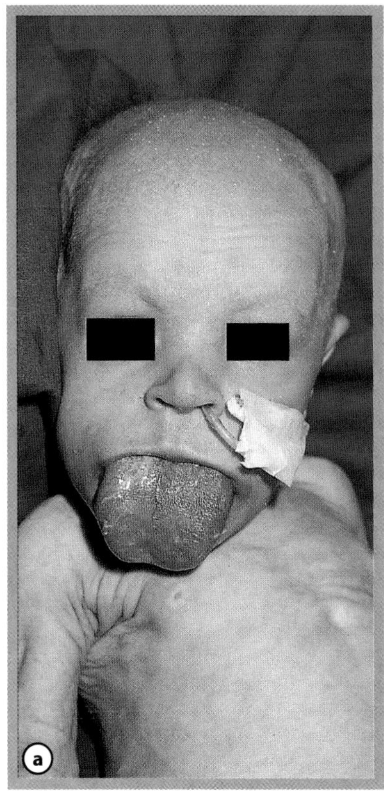

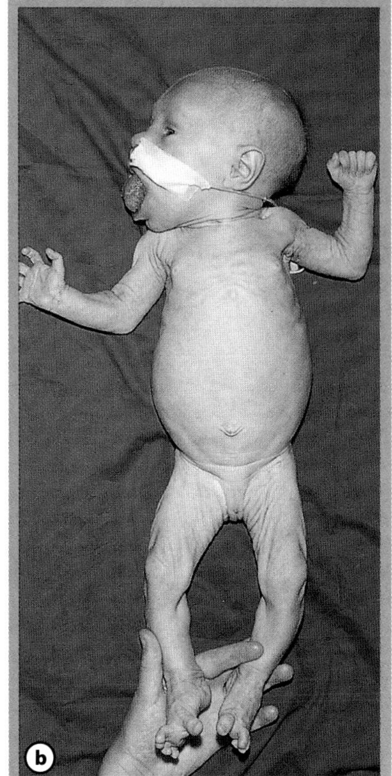

5.32a and 5.32b Macroglossia
An isolated case of macroglossia is shown, although it is often associated with conditions, for example, Beckwith–Wiedemann syndrome and hypothyroidism. The tongue may also be infiltrated by a haemangioma causing it to become enlarged. Feeding and respiratory difficulties may ensue and surgical resection of part of the tongue may be necessary.

6 Neurology

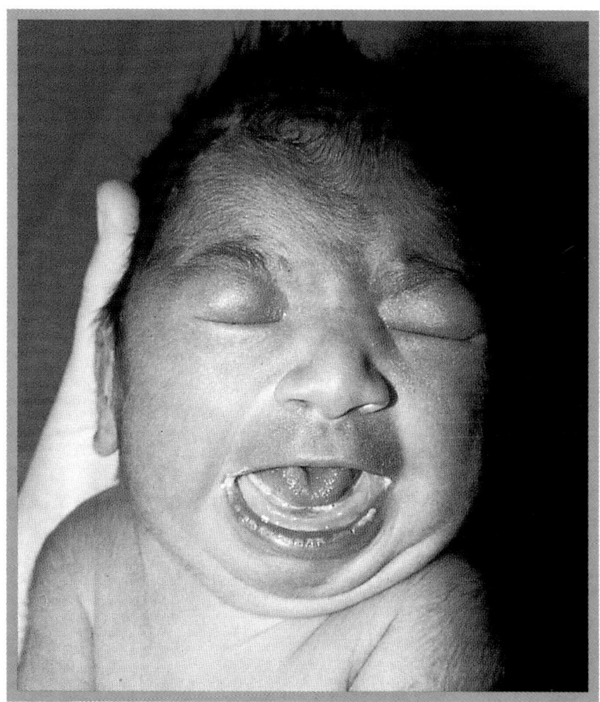

6.1 Microcephaly
The skull grows to accommodate the growing brain. If the brain is severely injured in any way, for example, infection such as maternal rubella, severe asphyxia or cerebral dysplasia, the final result will be microcephaly. This infant had congenital rubella and was later found to have severe mental retardation.

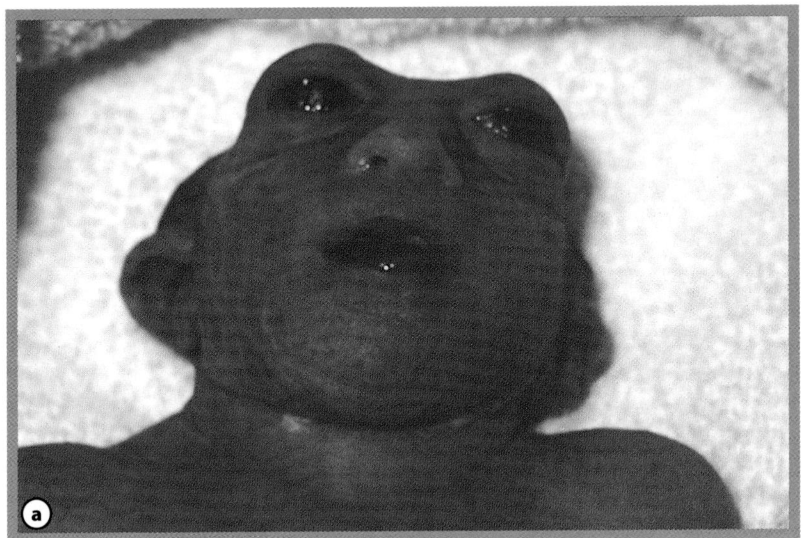

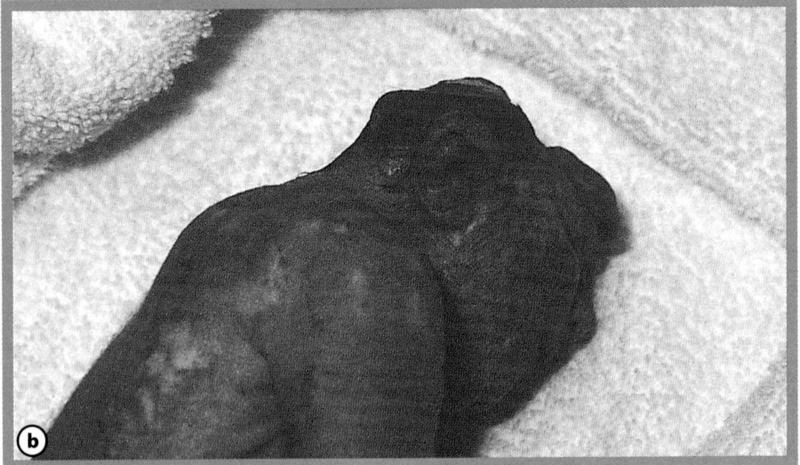

6.2a and 6.2b Anencephaly
This is the most severe neural tube defect with absent cerebral hemispheres incompatible with life. Rarely seen now due to antenatal detection and termination.

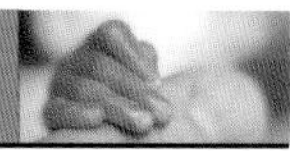

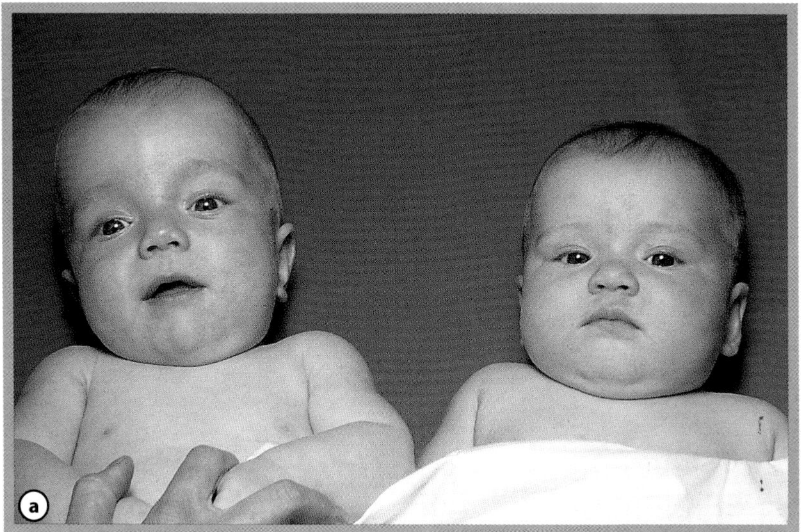

6.3a and 6.3b Post-haemorrhagic hydrocephalus
Twins who were born preterm are shown with one suffering from hydrocephalus caused by intra-ventricular haemorrhage. The setting sun sign is visible. Other causes include congenital aqueduct stenosis (*see* **6.4**), Arnold–Chiari malformation and neonatal meningitis.

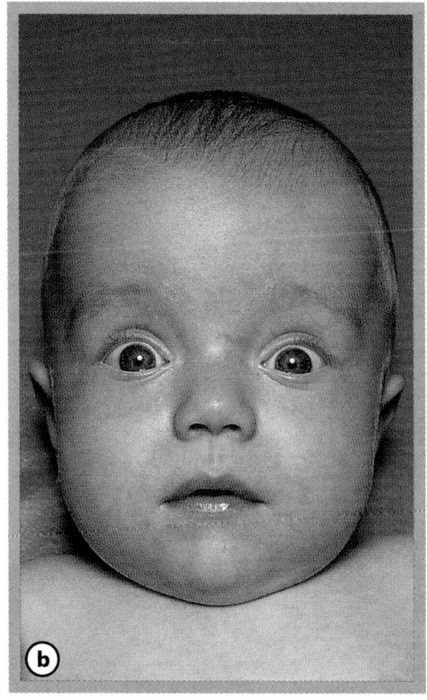

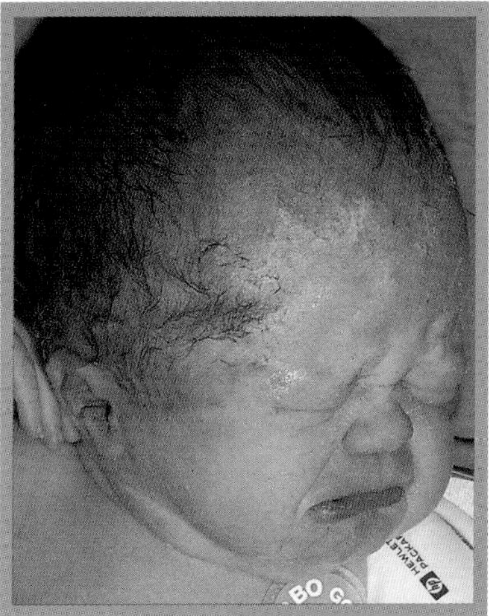

6.4 Congenital aqueduct stenosis

The infant shown has been delivered by elective caesarean section in view of the potential risk from a vaginal delivery. In this condition, the aetiology of which is unknown in the majority of patients, the aqueduct of Sylvius is either narrowed or forked at its distal end. A magnetic resonance imaging scan usually demonstrates the lesion.

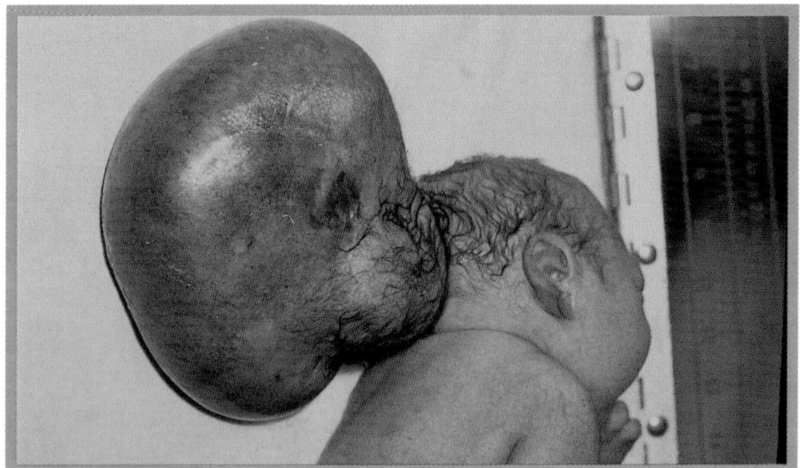

6.5 Encephalocoele

An extensive encephalocoele is seen, with the sac arising from the occiput containing brain tissue, thus differentiating the lesion from a cranial meningocoele in which the sac contains only cerebrospinal fluid. Frontal encephalocoeles are more common but when small, they may cause diagnostic confusion.

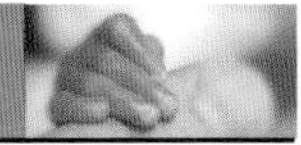

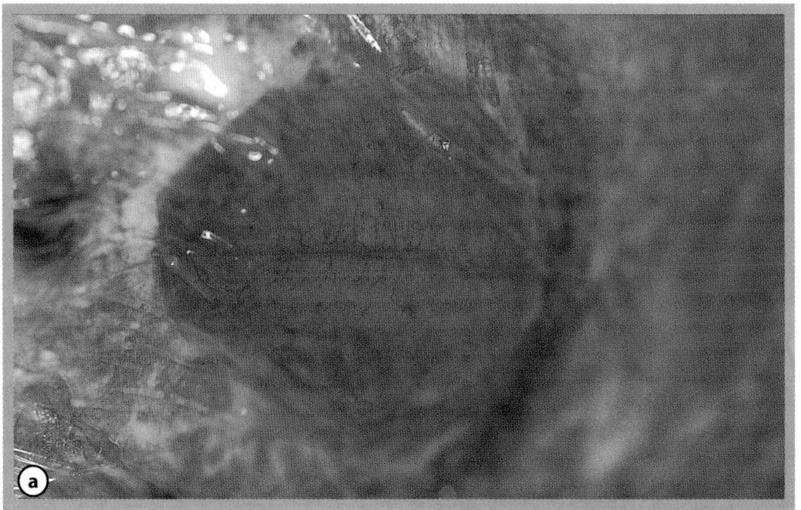

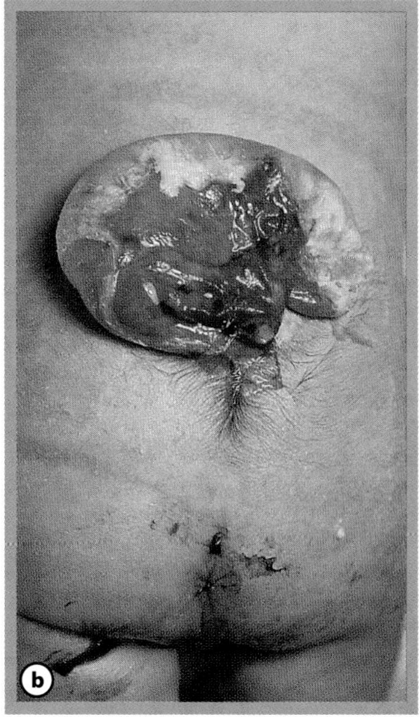

6.6a and 6.6b Spina bifida

The figure shows two infants with extensive thoracolumbar myelomeningocoeles with the exposed, poorly developed spinal cord, the neural plaque, clearly visible (**6.6a**). In order to protect the spinal cord the lesion was covered with cling film. The infant illustrated in **6.6b** has a patulous anus with the passage of meconium evident. This form of spina bifida carries the worst prognosis with likely complete paralysis of legs, anal and urethral incontinence, hydrocephalus, kyphosis and associated vesico-ureteric reflux.

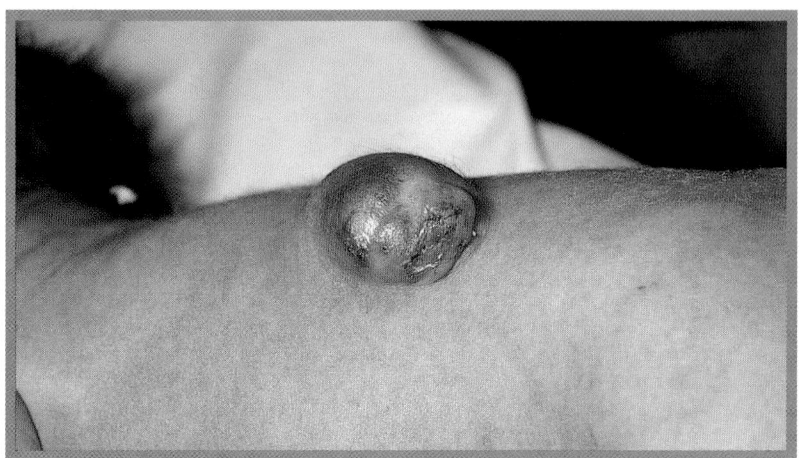

6.7 Thoracic meningomyelocoele
A limited meningomyelocoele is seen arising from the mid-thoracic region.

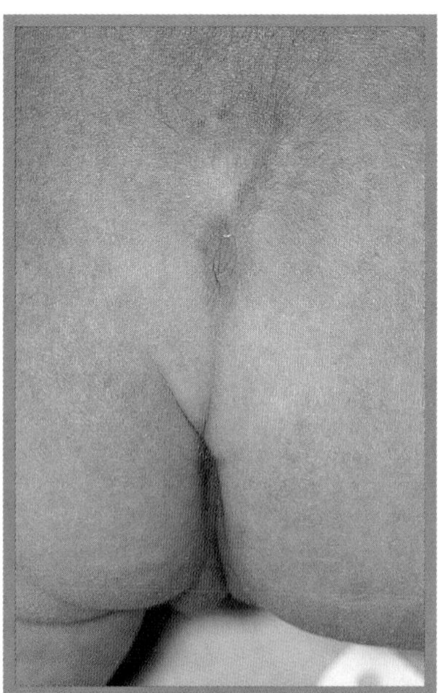

6.8 Spina bifida occulta
A hairy tuft with a small naevus is an outward sign of an underlying spina bifida occulta. Neurological abnormalities may occur in patients with overlying skin changes compared with patients with only incidental radiographic evidence of the vertebral defect. The condition is very common among the normal population.

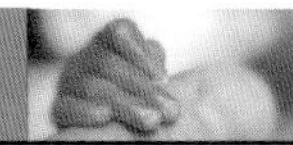

6.9a and 6.9b Hypotonic infant

This infant shows features of marked hypotonia with head lag and a frog-leg posture in the supine position. The causes may be classified as **central**, e.g. congenital cerebral malformations, or **peripheral**, e.g. anterior horn cell degeneration (Werdnig–Hoffman). In addition, numerous conditions and syndromes, e.g. hypothyroidism, Down syndrome, rickets, inborn errors and others, are associated with hypotonia.

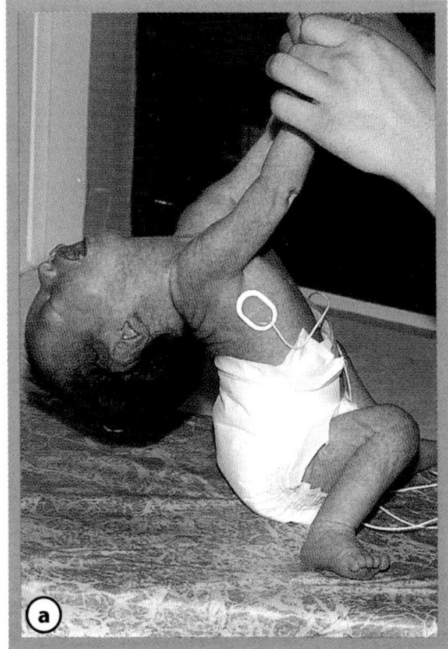

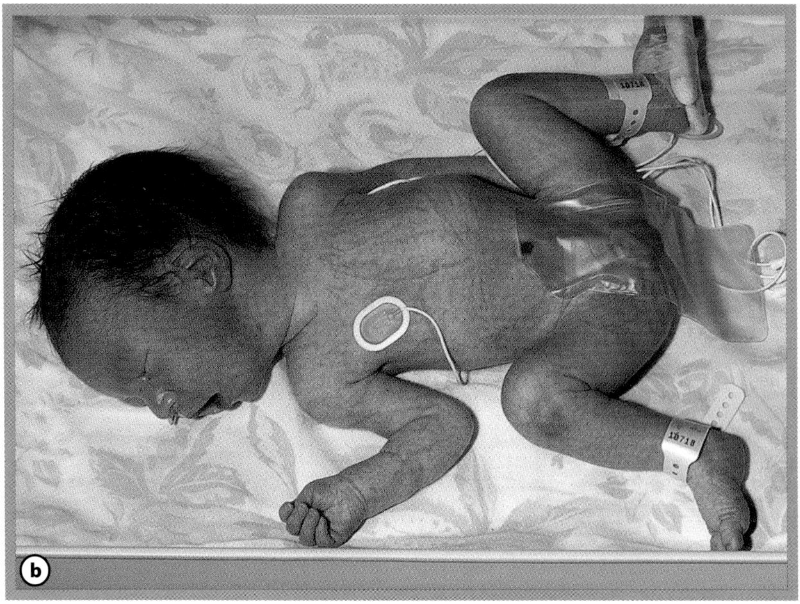

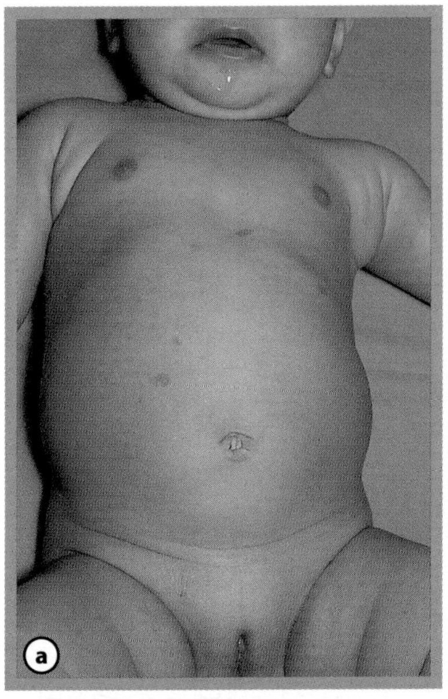

6.10a 6.10b and 6.10c Neurofibromatosis type I
This infant shows numerous café au lait spots. The diagnosis of type I neurofibromatosis was based on the association of the skin lesions and a first-degree relative with type I neurofibromatosis. Neurological complications may arise, including optic gliomas, meningiomas and spinal cord tumours. However, the expression of this condition may remain confined entirely to the skin. Axillary freckling, which as shown in this infant, commonly develops in mid-childhood.

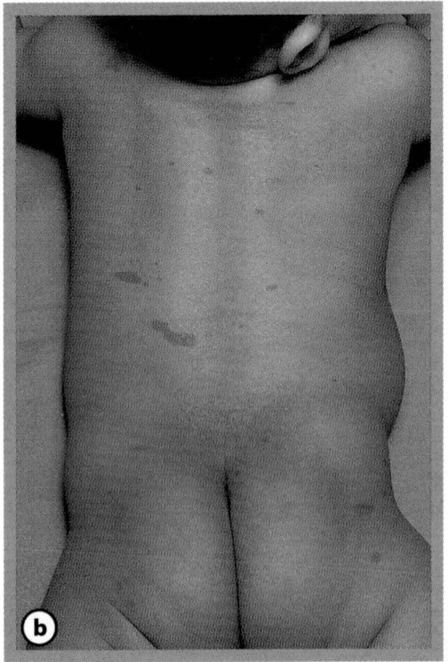

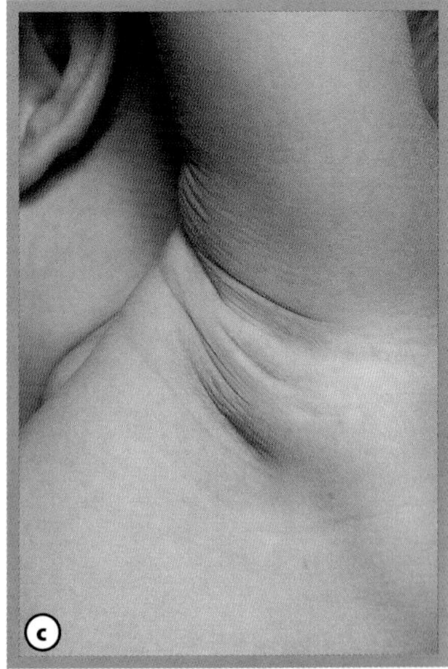

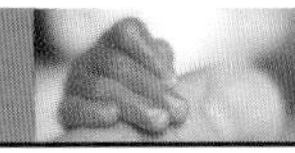

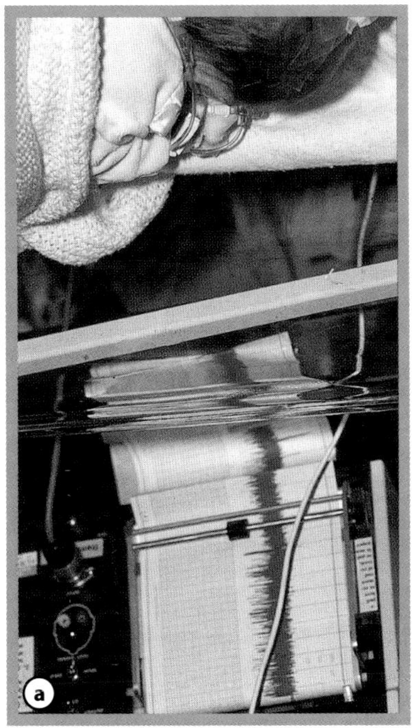

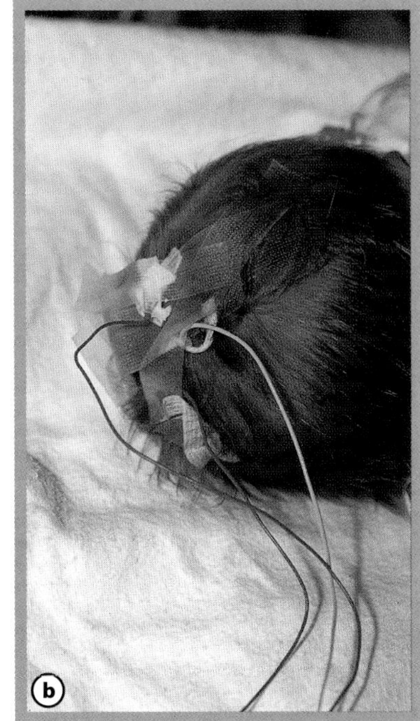

6.11a and 6.11b Cerebral function monitor

Cerebral function monitoring has been shown to be a valuable and reliable method for detecting abnormal brain activity at the bedside. Cerebral function recording is on a single channel electroencephalogram from two biparietal electrodes. The filtered signal is rectified, smoothed and the amplitude integrated and then written out at slow speed (6 cm/h). The resultant trace can be graded as abnormal if any of the following are present: burst-suppression, continuous low voltage or flat trace. In addition seizure activity can be clearly demonstrated.

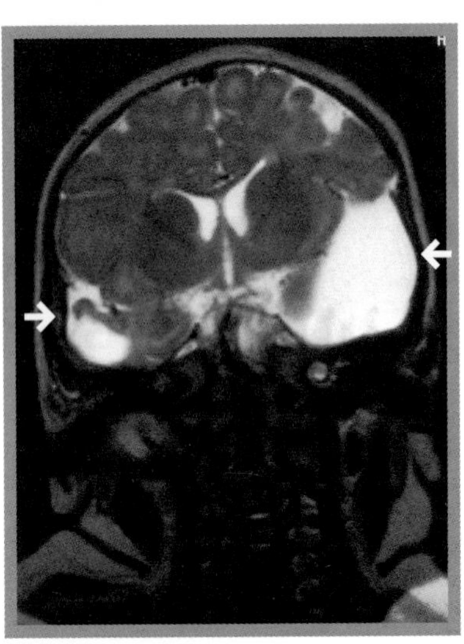

6.12 Congenital arachnoid cyst
This infant presented with fits. A coronal T_2-weighted magnetic resonance imaging scan shows bilateral middle cranial fossa arachnoid cysts. The left cyst is exerting some mass effect compressing the residual left temporal horn. Presentation of this condition with headache, hemiparesis, seizures or ataxia can occur at any time during life. Many of these cysts are, however, discovered at autopsy as an incidental finding.

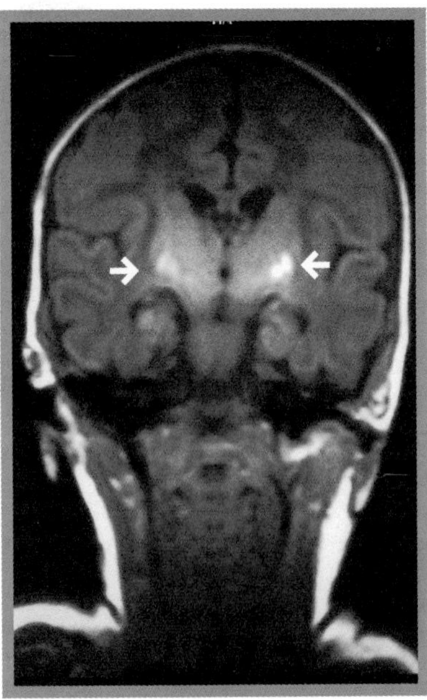

6.13 Hypoxic ischaemic damage to basal ganglia
This infant was born after an uneventful labour. At birth he had Apgar scores of 1, 4 and 6 at 1, 5 and 20 minutes respectively. The cause of his poor state at delivery remains unknown. The coronal T_1-weighted magnetic resonance imaging scan, carried out at 3 weeks of age, shows increased signals within both lentiform nuclei. Clinically, the infant exhibited evidence of moderately severe motor dysfunction.

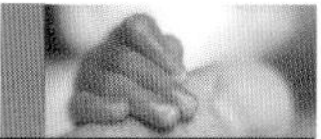

6.14 Agenesis of the corpus collosum

This infant presented with gross hypotonia and was found to have duplication of the short arm of chromosome 8. The coronal T_1-weighted magnetic resonance imaging scan shows agenesis of the corpus collosum and hemiatrophy of the left cerebral hemisphere. Agenesis of the corpus collosum has increasingly been associated with other central nervous system abnormalities.

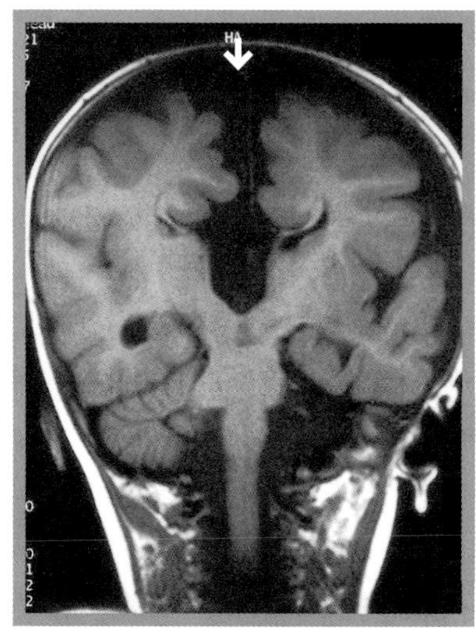

6.15 Multiple cysts secondary to perinatal intra-ventricular haemorrhages and ischaemia

This premature infant (24-weeks gestation) had multiple intra-ventricular bleeds with associated parenchymal infarcts. The coronal T_1-weighted magnetic resonance imaging scan shows bilateral ventricular enlargement as a result of white matter atrophy. On the right side there are large cerebrospinal fluid spaces within the brain parenchyma at the site of the previous haemorrhages. Clinically, this infant has significant motor and cognitive impairment.

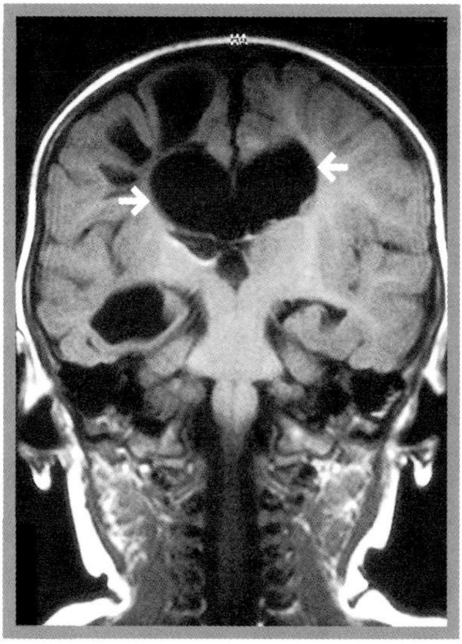

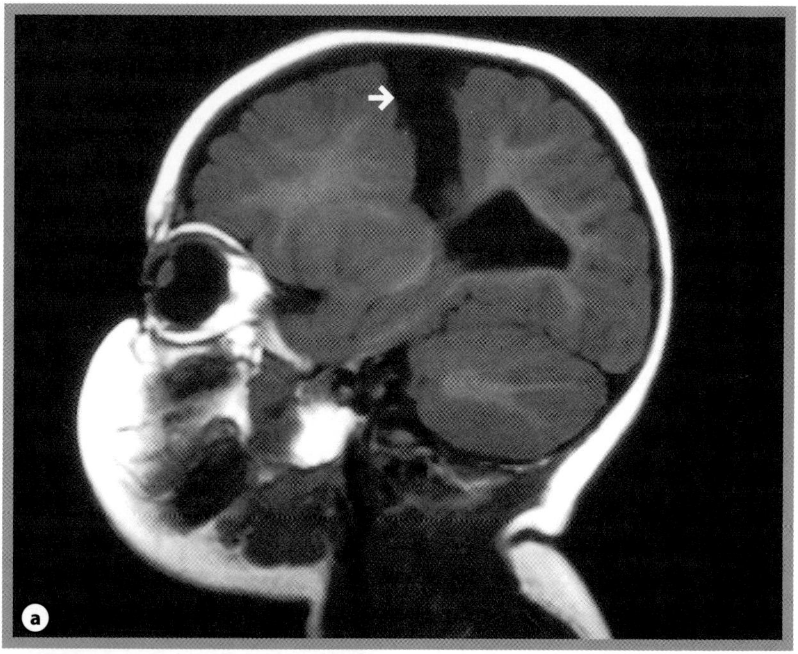

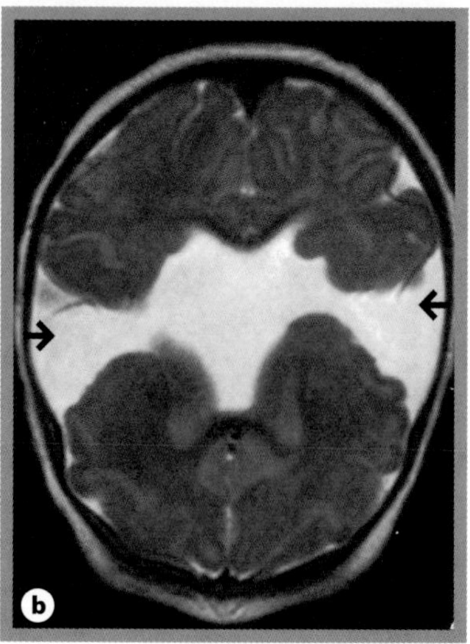

6.16a and 6.16b Bilateral open-lipped schizencephaly
This infant presented with microcephaly and developmental delay. The figures show an axial T_1-weighted (**6.16a**) and a parasaggital T_1-weighted (**6.16b**) magnetic resonance imaging scan. They show bilateral cerebrospinal fluid-filled cysts extending from the cortex to the lateral ventricles. Note the cleft is lined with grey matter. This condition is rare and usually occurs as a result of an environmental insult during early gestation.

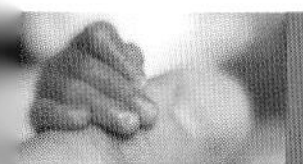

7 Cardiothoracic

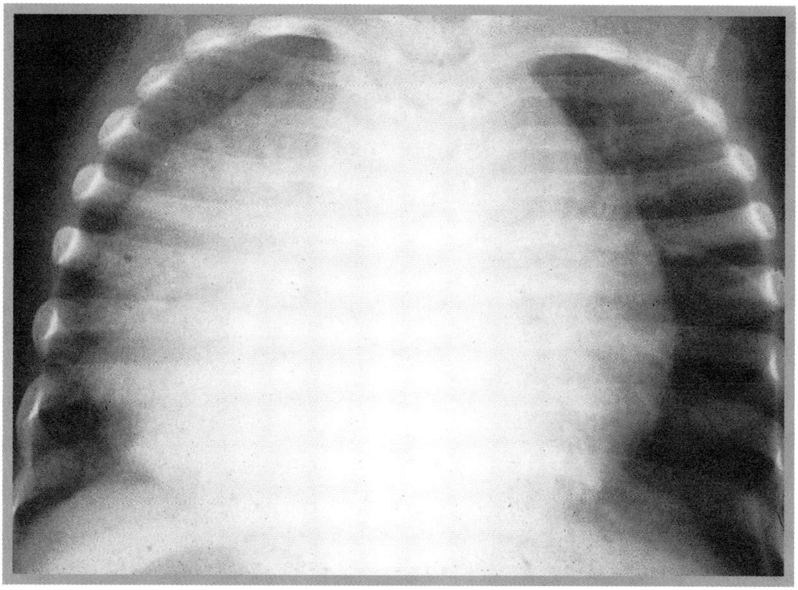

7.1 Pericardial effusion

Pericardial effusions are uncommon in neonatology; they may be infective; iatrogenic, usually secondary to a long line placement; or of unknown aetiology. In this infant no cause was found. The effusion did not compromise cardiac function and resolved without intervention.

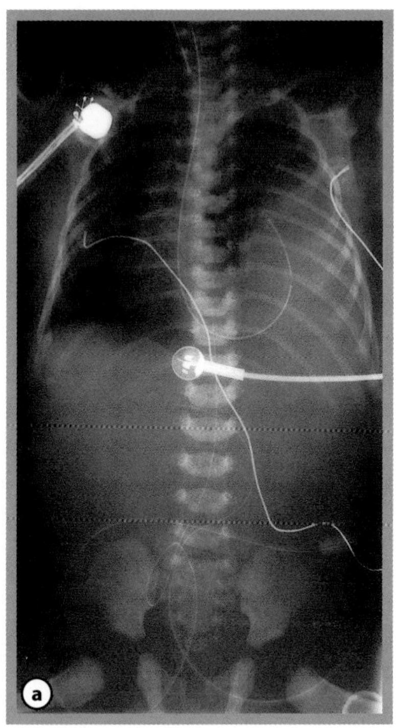

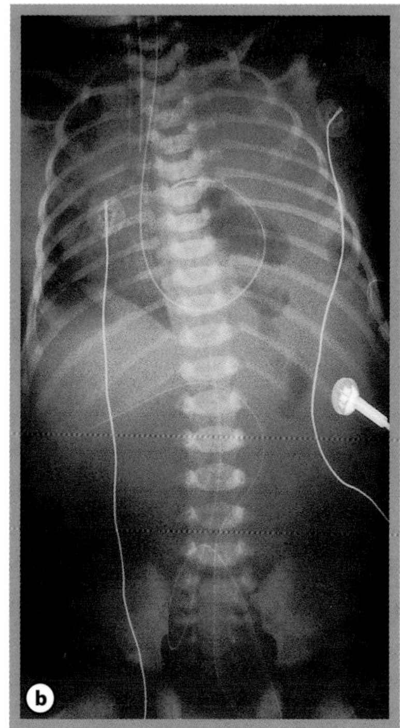

7.2a, 7.2b and 7.2c Diaphragmatic hernia

At 1 hour of age before any swallowed air reached the bowel (**7.2a**), the nasogastric tube was curled up in the stomach, which was displaced into the thoracic cavity. Air in the stomach and small bowel is shown in **7.2b**. In addition paucity of air in the abdomen is seen. Resuscitation of this premature infant was impossible: the autopsy clearly shows the abdominal contents within the thoracic cavity (**7.2c**).

This condition occurs relatively commonly in about 1 out of 3000 deliveries. As a result of a defect in the formation of the diaphragm within the first 8 weeks of gestation, the abdominal contents are able to enter the thoracic cavity. This leads to various degrees of lung hypoplasia. Most diaphragmatic hernias are now diagnosed antenatally. Delivery should be planned in a neonatal unit with paediatric surgeons in attendance. The mainstay of treatment is initial stabilization and subsequent surgery. Prognosis is good if the infant can be adequately stabilized.

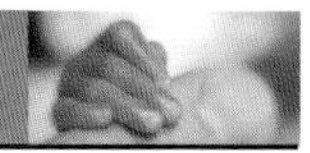

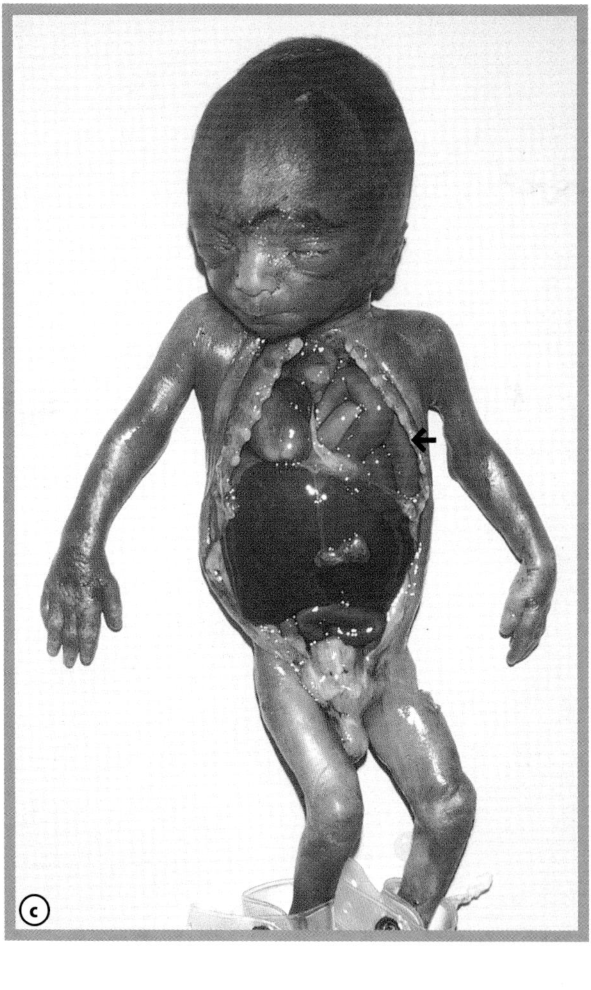

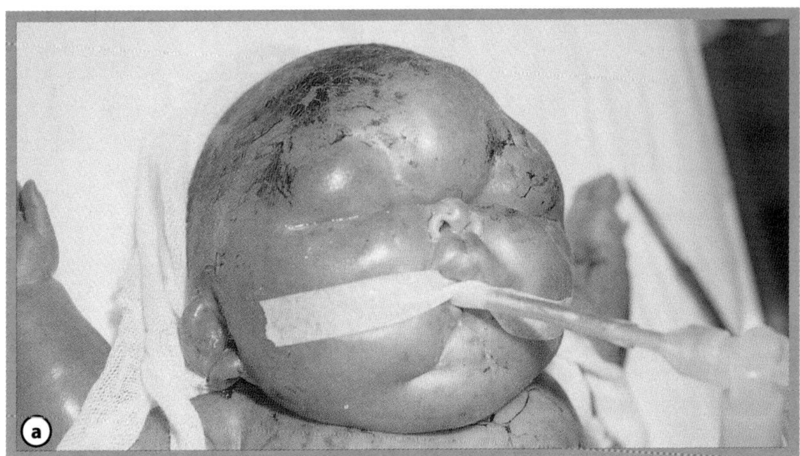

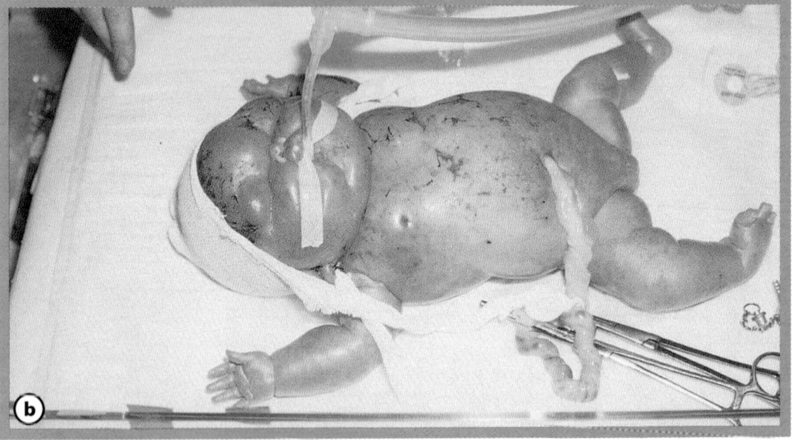

7.3a and 7.3b Hydrops foetalis

The incidence of hydrops has dramatically decreased in recent times because of the use of rhesus immunoglobulin and antenatal transfusions. Two types of hydrops have been recognized:

1. Immune, caused by maternal isoimmunization against either rhesus or other red cell antigens.
2. Non-immune, due to other ill-defined mechanisms.

The infant in this figure had immune hydrops secondary to rhesus disease.

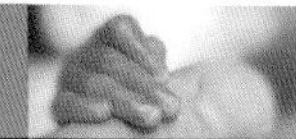

7.4 Cyanotic infant

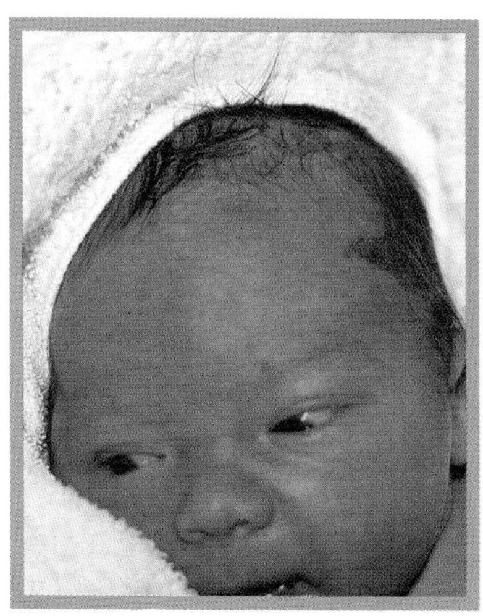

Cyanosis in the neonate is common. There are three main causes of cyanosis:

1. Poor tissue perfusion with no underlying cardiac or respiratory problem.
2. Respiratory.
3. Cardiac.

This infant was aged 4 hour and had transposition of the great arteries. His oxygen saturation was 20%, which did not change when given 100% inspired oxygen (nitrogen wash-out test). After corrective surgery he made a complete recovery.

7.5 Fallot's tetralogy

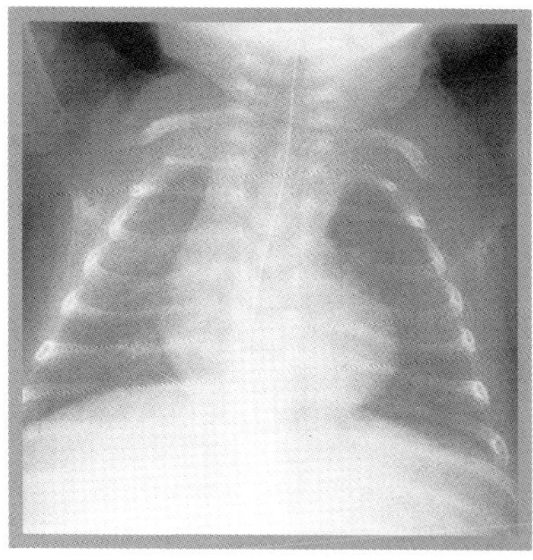

This radiograph shows the up-tilted cardiac apex (boot-shaped heart). In severe Fallot's, the lung fields are usually oligaemic. A right-sided aortic arch is seen in 20% of patients. This infant presented with a murmur at the age of 4 weeks.

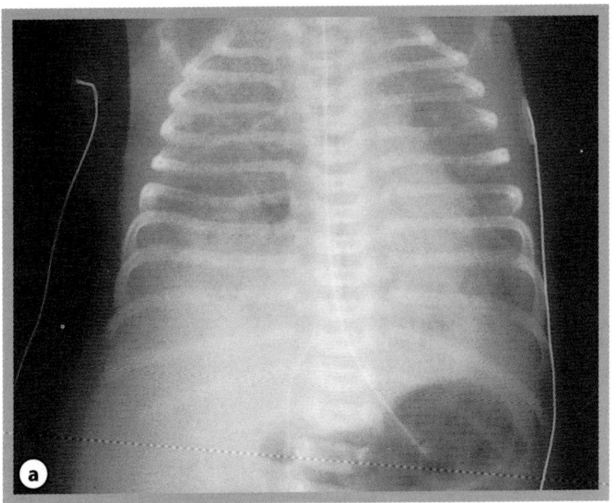

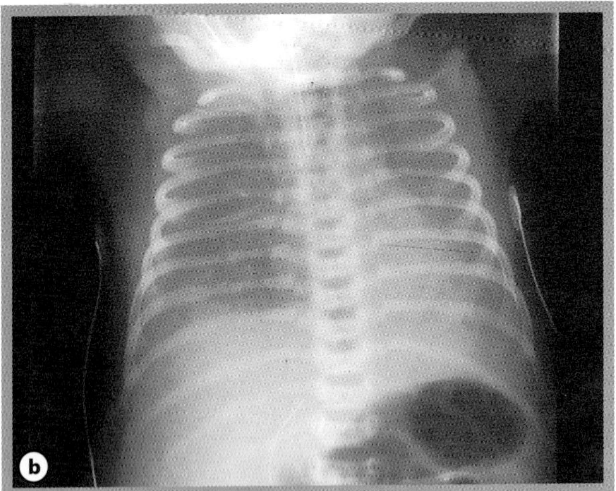

7.6a, 7.6b, 7.6c and 7.6d Congenital pneumonia (group β streptococcal pneumonia)

The first radiograph was taken at 4 hours of age in this term infant. The only clinical finding initially was mild recession. The infant soon deteriorated and needed ventilation. Antibiotics were started at the age of 4 hours. The subsequent two films were taken at days 2 and 7, respectively. Group β

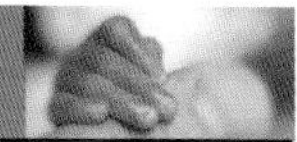

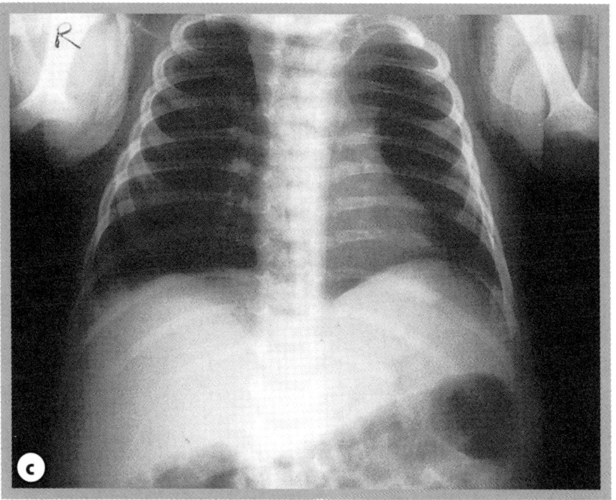

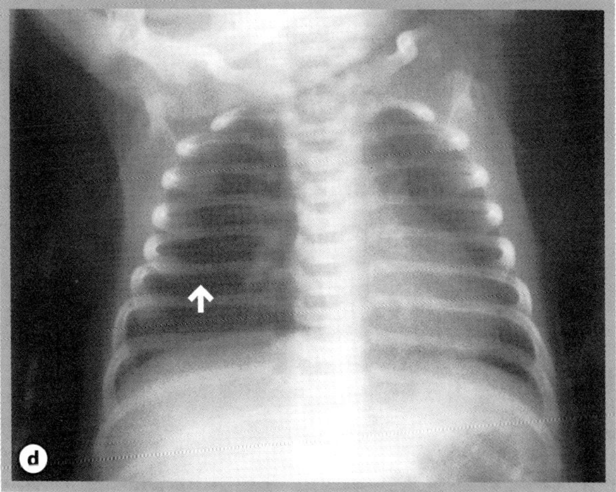

streptococcus was isolated from blood cultures.

The infant shown in **7.6d** collapsed in the post-natal ward aged 2 days. Note the fluid in the horizontal fissure which may be the only clue to the possible presence of group β streptococcal sepsis (which was in fact isolated from the blood cultures after 24 hours). This infant died from overwhelming sepsis after being ventilated for 2 days.

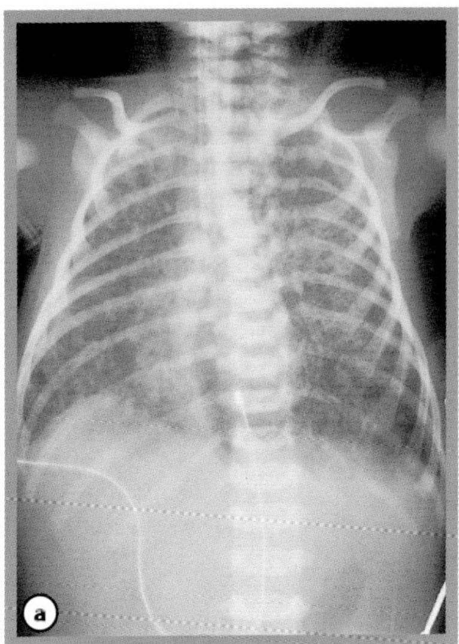

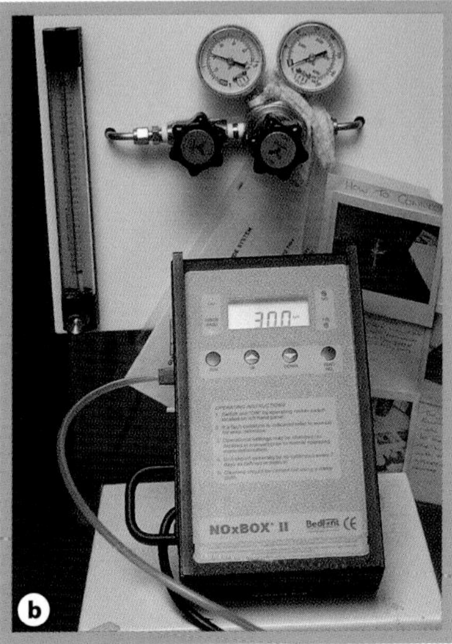
NOxBOX II
Bedfont

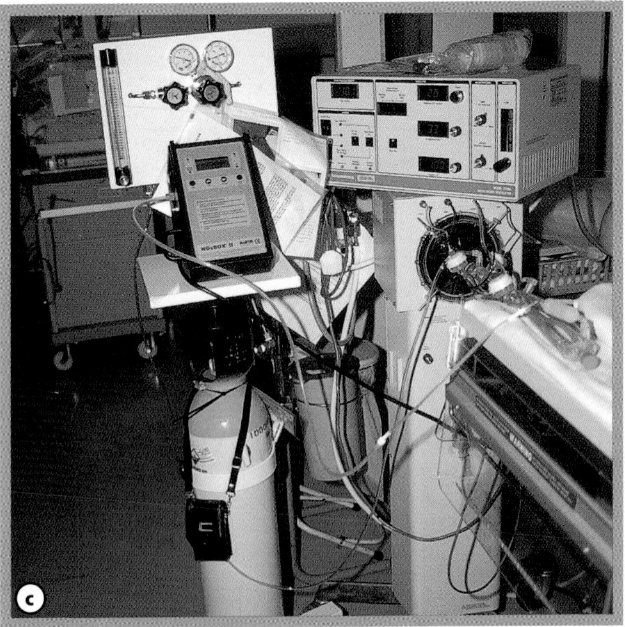

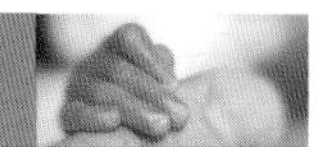

7.7a, 7.7b and 7.7c Meconium aspiration

Meconium aspiration occurs as a result of inhalation of meconium passed *in utero*. The precise mechanism responsible for aspiration of meconium is still unclear. However, it is mostly associated with intra-partum ischaemic events. The characteristic radiograph findings, as shown in **7.7a** are bilateral patchy coarse shadowing with associated hyperinflation. Management is often difficult, in order to avoid excess ventilator-related volume trauma, new strategies including high-frequency oscillation (**7.7c**) have been developed. Nitric oxide is often used to treat the associated pulmonary hypertension (**7.7b**). However recent trials have cast some doubt on this therapy.

7.8 Tracheo-oesophageal fistula and oesophageal atresia

This figure shows a contrast study that demonstrates oesophageal atresia and a tracheo-oesophageal fistula. Contrast passes through the fistula, outlining the bronchial tree and the distal oesophagus and stomach, confirming the presence of an H-type fistula.

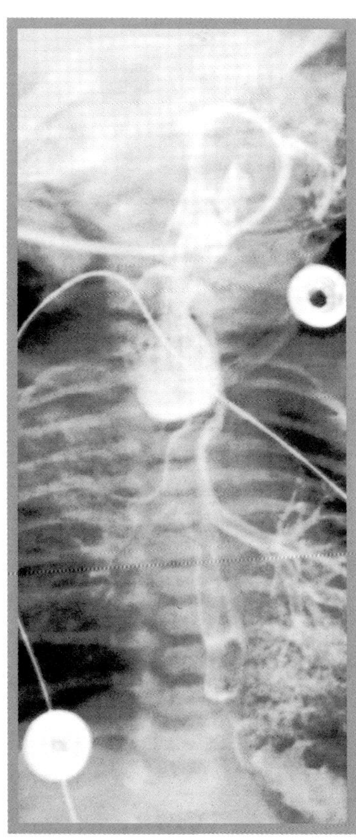

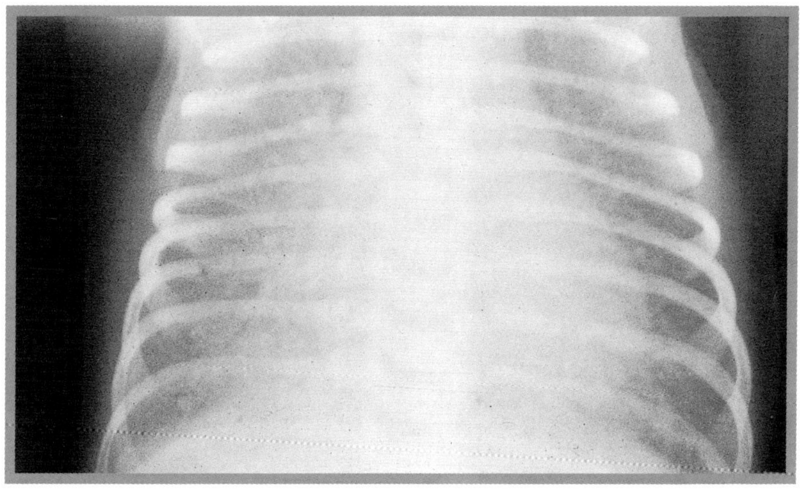

7.9 Total anomalous pulmonary venous drainage obstruction
This condition is a rare cause of cyanosis and respiratory distress in the newborn. Obstruction of the pulmonary venous return, due to abnormal venous drainage, leads to intensely congested lungs and pulmonary oedema as shown in the chest radiograph. Infants presenting in the neonatal period require early surgery.

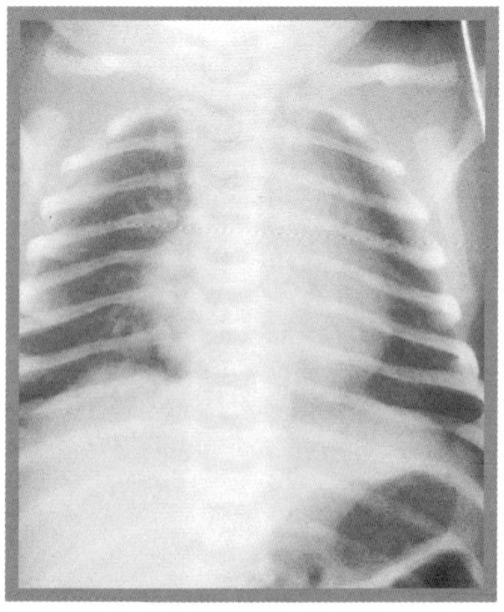

7.10 Transient tachypnoea of the newborn
This term infant's respiratory rate was 120/min, blood cultures were negative and he recovered after 72 hours. The chest radiograph shows fluid in the horizontal fissure. This condition is thought to arise from delayed clearance of lung fluid. It is more common in term infants who classically present with tachypnoea. There are generally no other signs of respiratory distress. The diagnosis is one of exclusion, as sepsis must be ruled out.

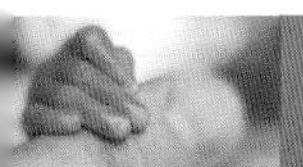

8 Gastrointestinal and genito-urinary

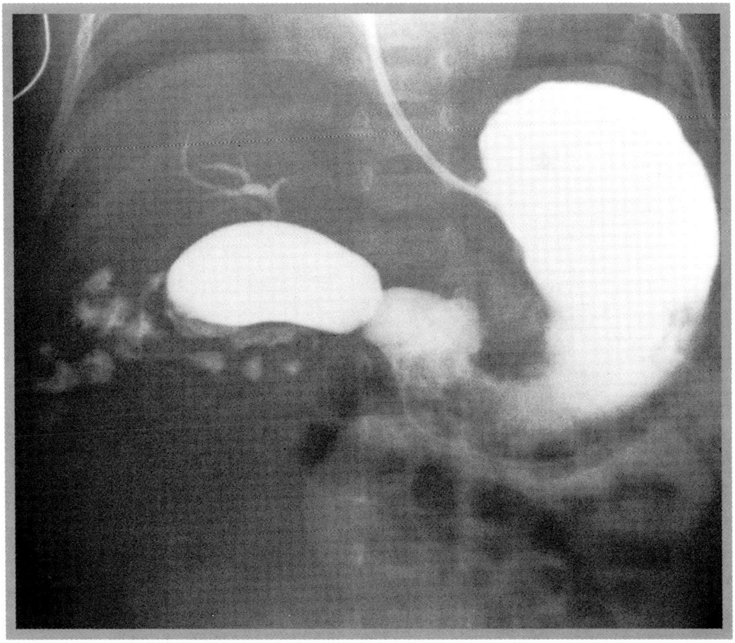

8.1 Duodenal web and malrotation

This barium study shows malrotation of the duodenum, as shown by contrast in the proximal jejunum lying to the right of the mid-line, with a defect secondary to a web at the duodenal loop. Affected infants usually present in the first 12 months of life with bile-stained vomiting caused by mid-gut volvulus. Chronic symptoms of vomiting may also be the presenting features and indeed some infants remain asymptomatic.

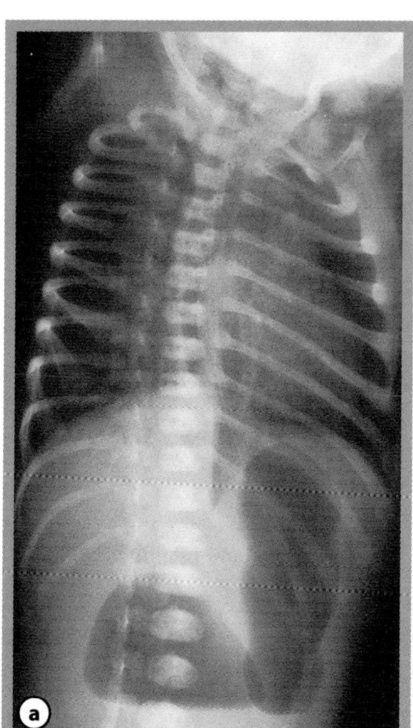

8.2a and 8.2b Duodenal atresia The classical double bubble associated with duodenal atresia is shown. The infant will usually present within the first few hours of life with bile-stained vomiting. Antenatal diagnosis is common, prompted by the presence of polyhydramnios and ultrasound findings of fluid-filled cysts in the foetal abdomen. The defect is strongly associated with Down syndrome. Surgical correction is indicated once the infant is stable. The atretic segment with proximal dilatation of the duodenum is clearly shown (**8.2b**).

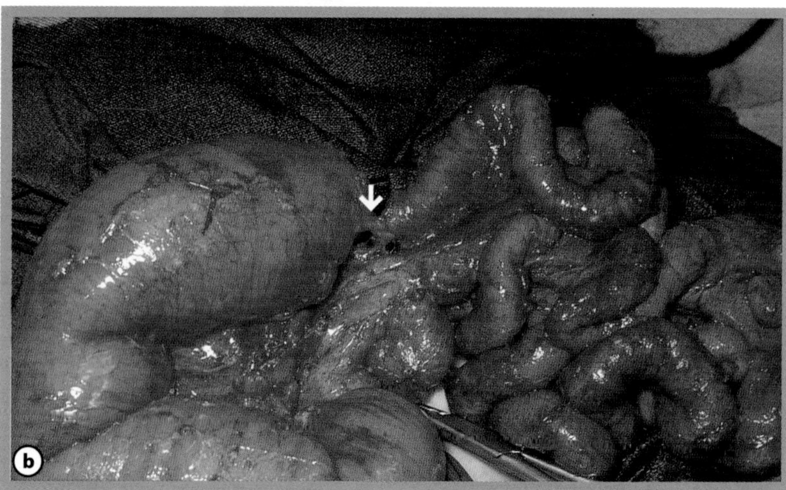

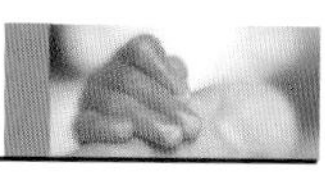

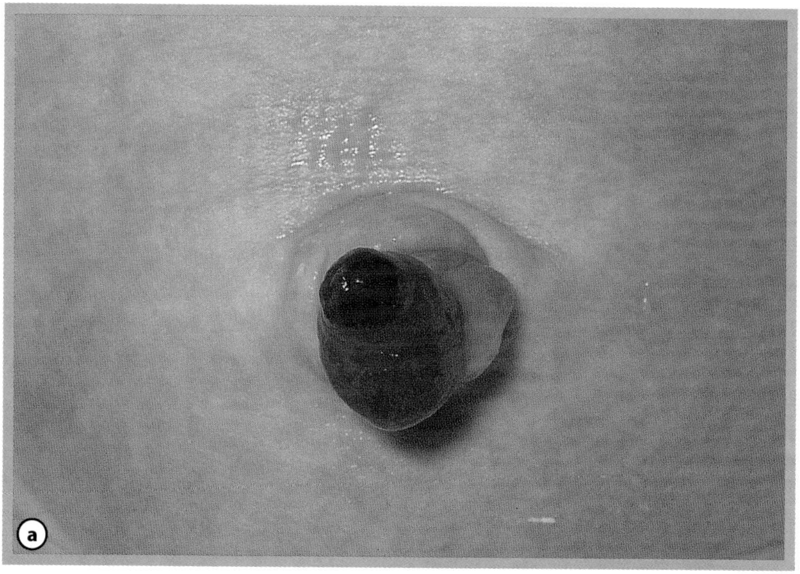

8.3a and 8.3b Persistence of vitello-intestinal duct

This embryological remnant is often confused with umbilical granuloma. The key to the diagnosis is the faeculent discharge that occurs, although this can be mistaken for a purulent discharge within an infected umbilicus. Contrast studies confirm the presence of the duct which is usually attached to the small intestine at the origin of a Meckel's diverticulum. A catheter is shown inserted into the duct (**8.3b**). It is important not to confuse this with an umbilical granuloma (*see* **8.7**).

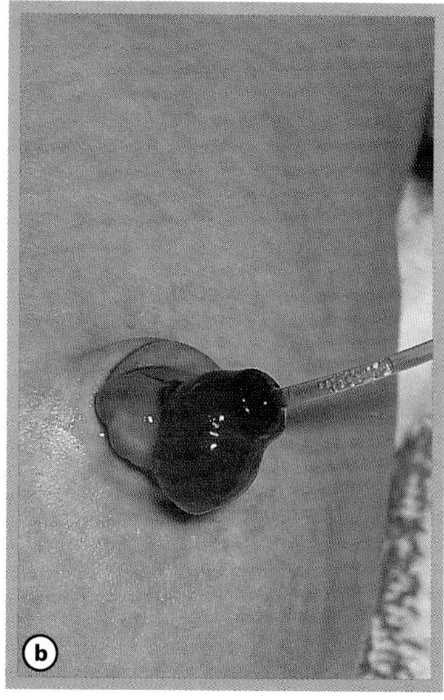

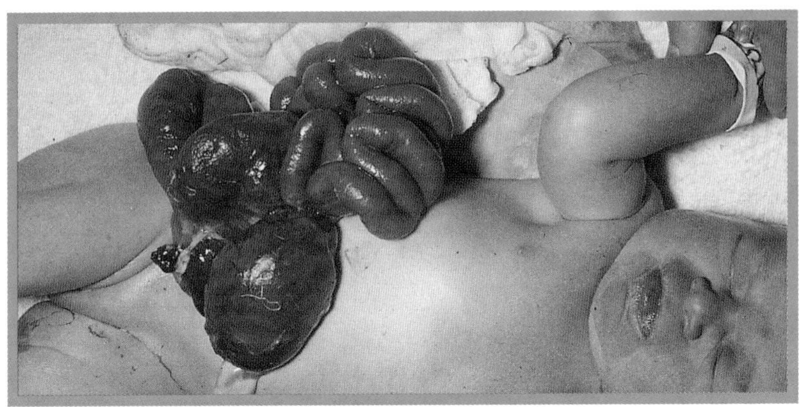

8.4 Gastroschisis
Gastroschisis is a developmental defect involving the abdominal wall, more commonly to the right of the umbilicus. The entire length of the intestine including the stomach may be extruded. Fluid loss may be extreme from the exposed small bowel after birth and the contents must be covered immediately in warm soaks. Replacement of the contents through the defect may be straightforward but may require a gradual approach as in exomphalos.

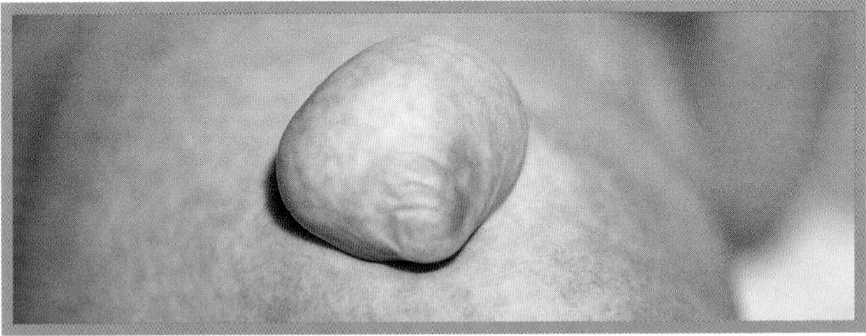

8.5 Umbilical hernia
Separation of the umbilical cord is normally associated with closure of the umbilical ring. In a proportion of children this fails to close completely, resulting in the defect shown. In most children the hernia closes of its own accord by the time the child is aged 2 years. If it persists beyond this period, surgical closure is usually required if only to stave off peer ridicule as strangulation is highly unlikely.

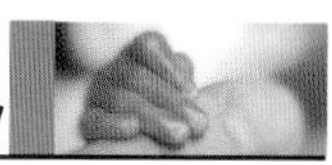

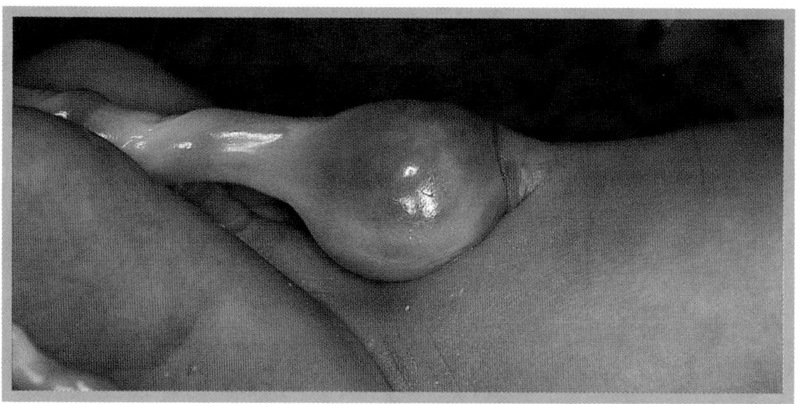

8.6 Herniation of umbilical cord

This represents herniation of the small bowel into the umbilicus as a result of a failure of the complete migration of the abdominal contents back into the abdominal cavity. It is the mildest end of the exomphalos or omphalocoele spectrum of disorders.

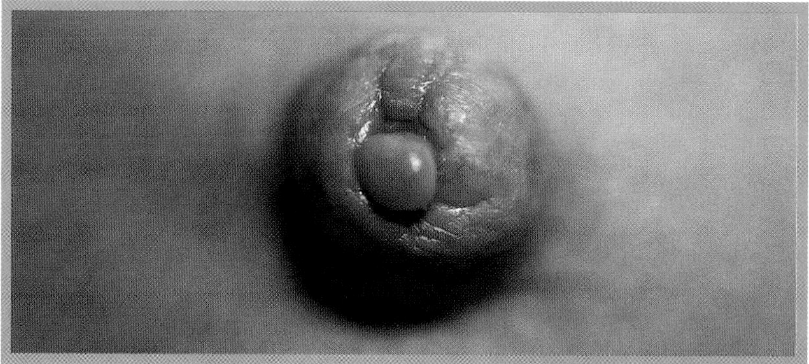

8.7 Umbilical granuloma

After separation of the umbilical cord the stump normally heals within 2 weeks. On occasions, however, granulation tissue remains at the base of the cord often causing a small amount of discharge. The most appropriate treatment is to apply silver nitrate to the granulation tissue taking care not to contaminate healthy surrounding tissue (*see* **14.7**).

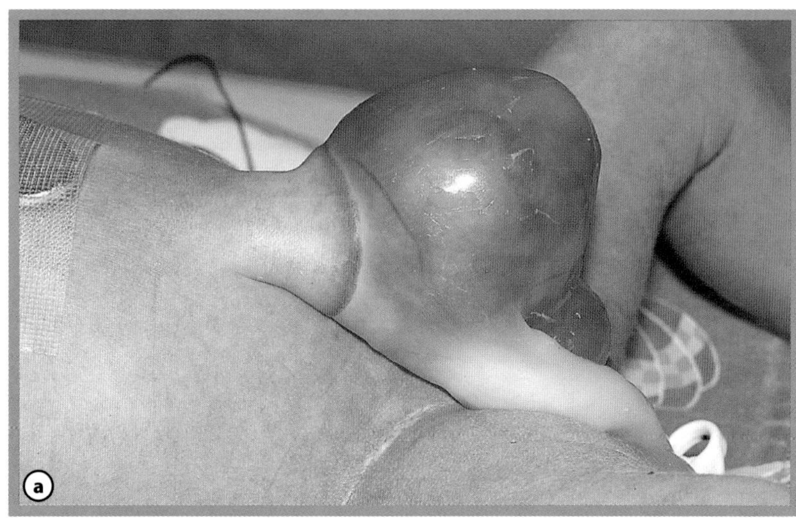

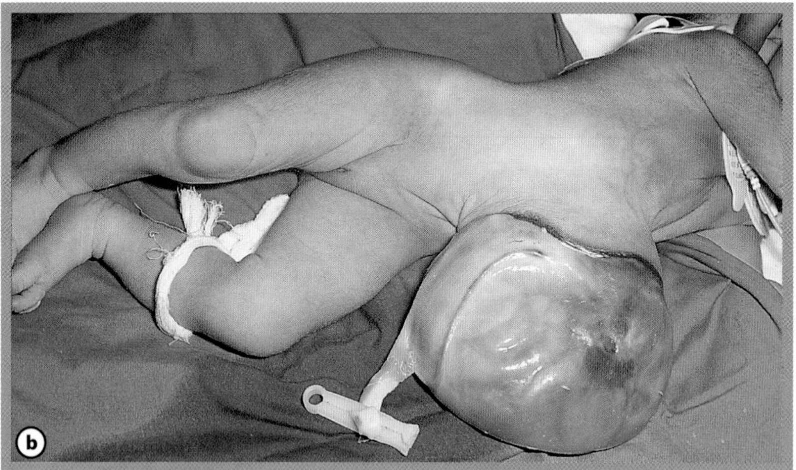

8.8a, 8.8b, 8.8c, 8.8d, 8.8e and 8.8f Exomphalos
Various degrees of true exomphalos are illustrated. The extruded sac contains bowel (**8.8a**) and in **8.8b** and **8.8c** liver is also contained in the sac. Other associated congenital abnormalities are common (e.g. renal anomalies). The management consists of initial application of cling film to protect the

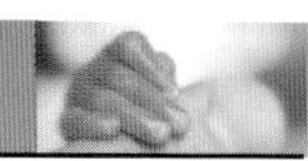

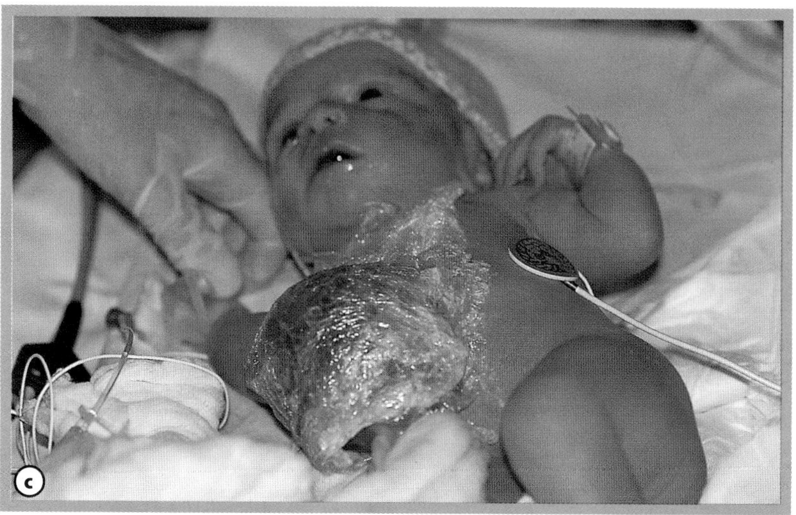

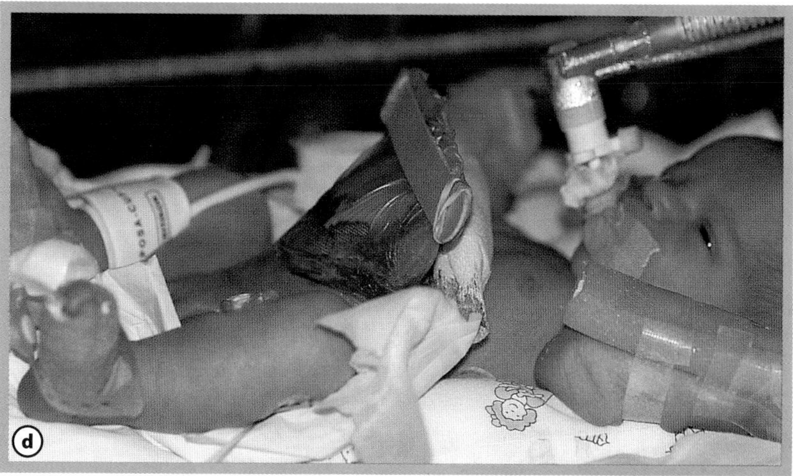

exteriorized bowel (**8.8c**) and then gradual reduction of the contents back into the abdominal cavity using a silastic pouch and spatula as shown (**8.8d** and **8.8e**). Subsequent closure of the abdominal defect can then be attempted. An excellent long-term outcome is shown (**8.8f**).

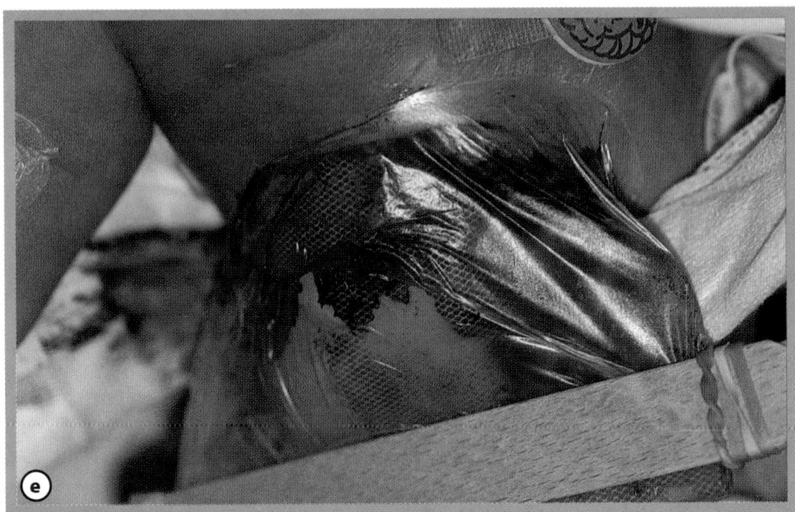

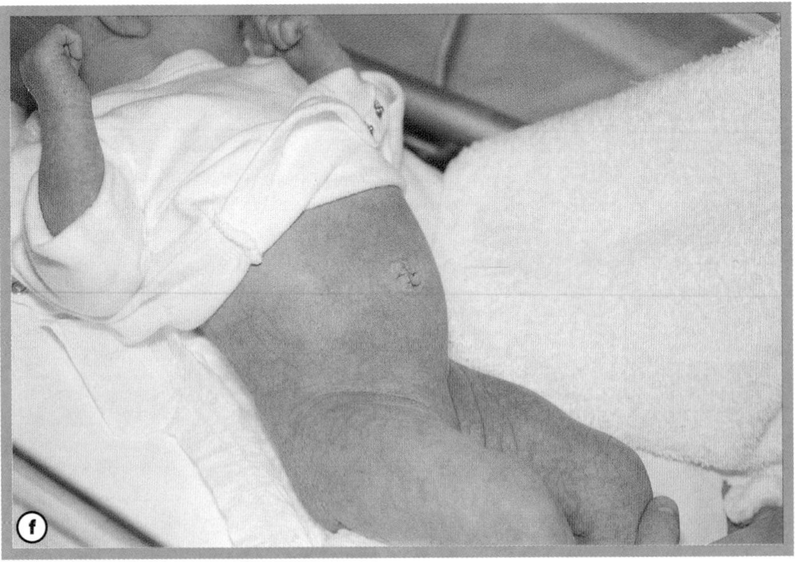

8.8e and 8.8f Exomphalos continued

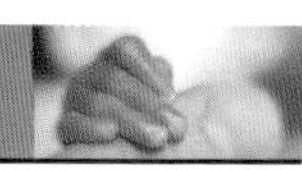

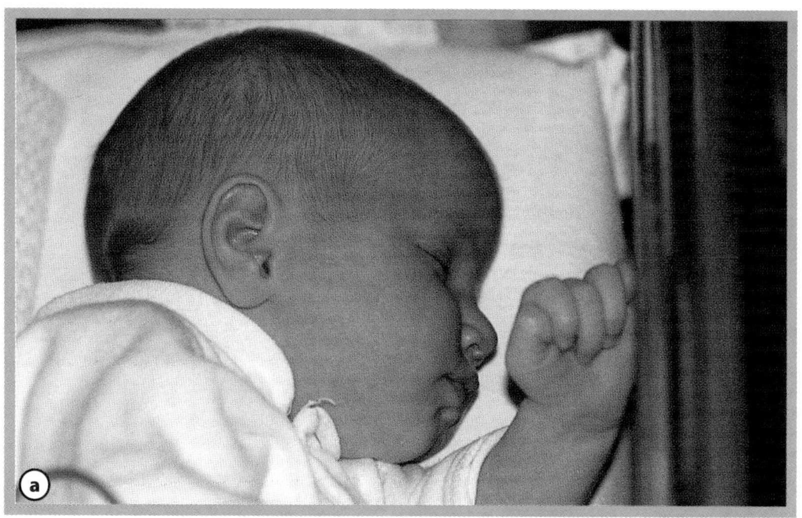

8.9a and 8.9b Conjugated jaundice

This shows the classical appearance with pale stools. Causes to be excluded include biliary atresia, biliary hypoplasia, choledochal cyst, infective and cryptogenic hepatitis and metabolic disorders (e.g. tyrosinaemia and alpha-1 anti-trypsin deficiency).

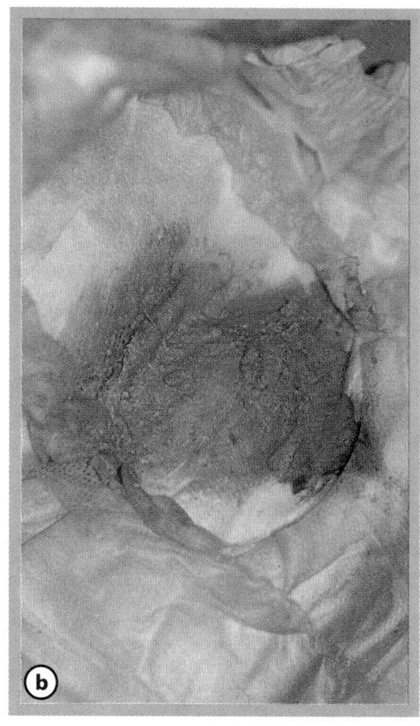

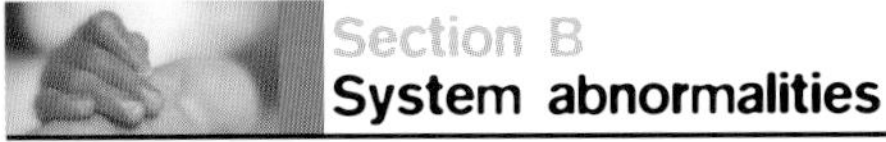

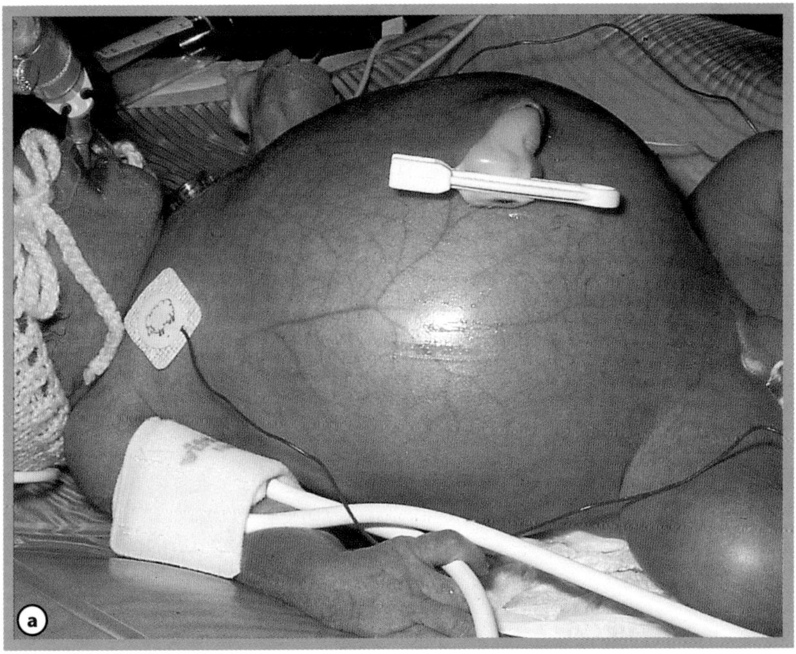

a

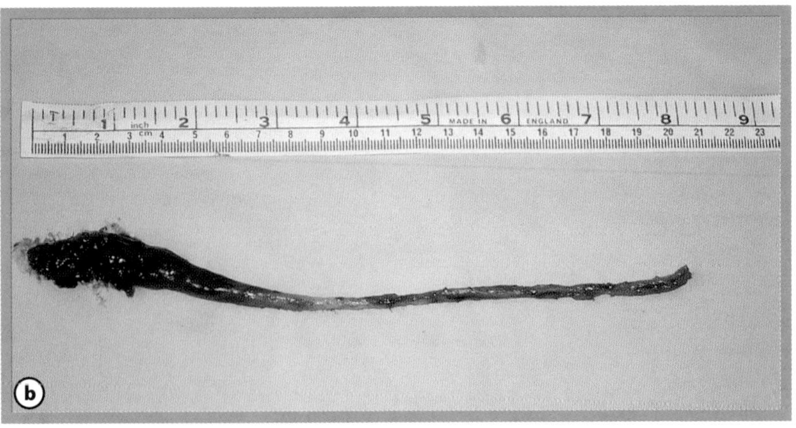

b

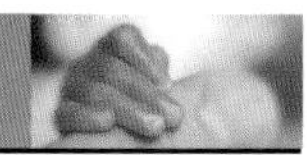

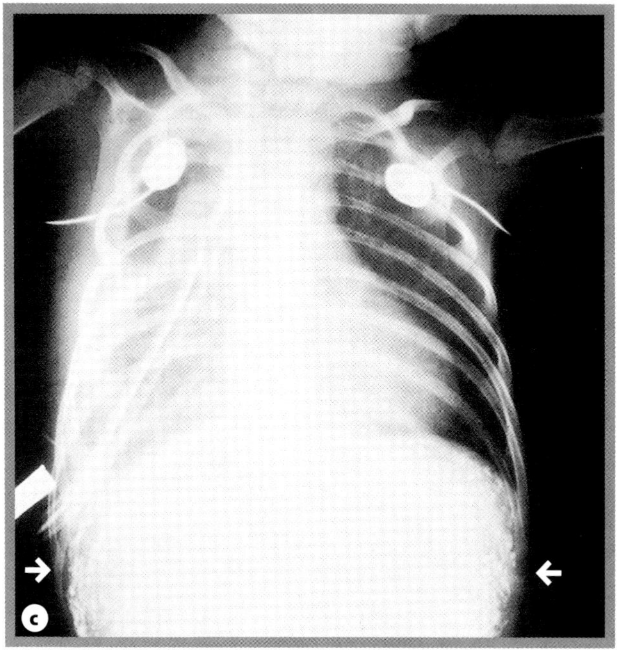

8.10a, 8.10b and 8.10c Meconium ileus
A markedly distended abdomen is shown with the cause clearly demonstrated. The extensive meconium plug was retrieved using a contrast enema (**8.10b**). Some patients require a formal laparotomy to clear the obstruction with direct lavage of the bowel. Antenatal bowel perforation may occur, resulting in peritoneal calcification (see arrows) as shown in **8.10c**. This patient also had a right-sided drain for meconium aspiration syndrome. A diagnosis of cystic fibrosis should be suspected for infants presenting with this condition.

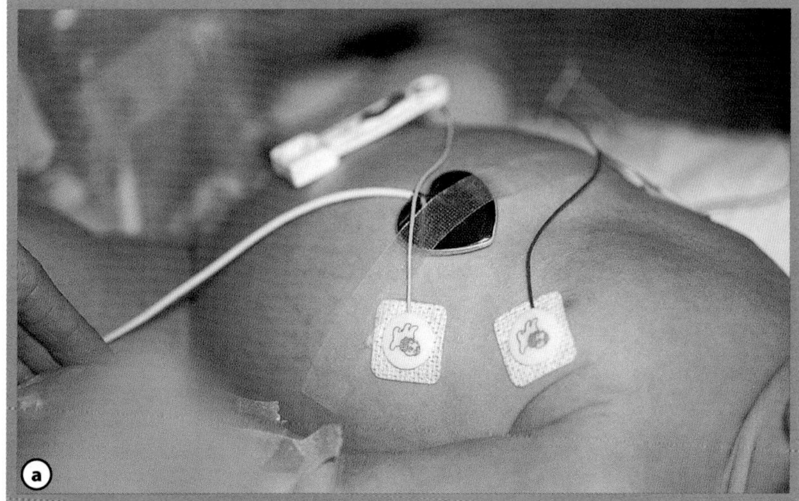

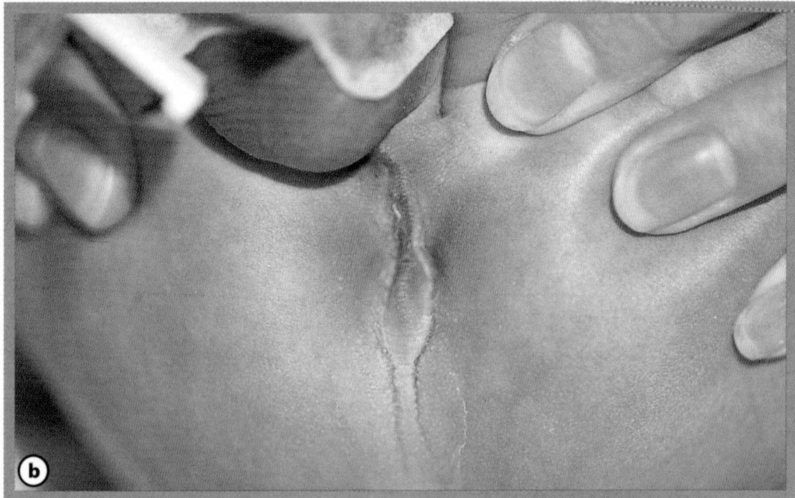

8.11a, 8.11b, 8.11c and 8.11d Anal stenosis with obstruction
This infant presented within 24 hours of birth with abdominal distension (**8.11a**) and bile-stained vomiting (**8.11c**). A complete anal stenosis can be seen (**8.11b**) and, in this infant, was associated with rectal agenesis, as suggested by the

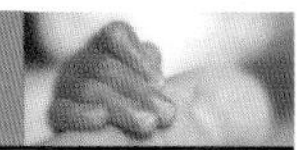

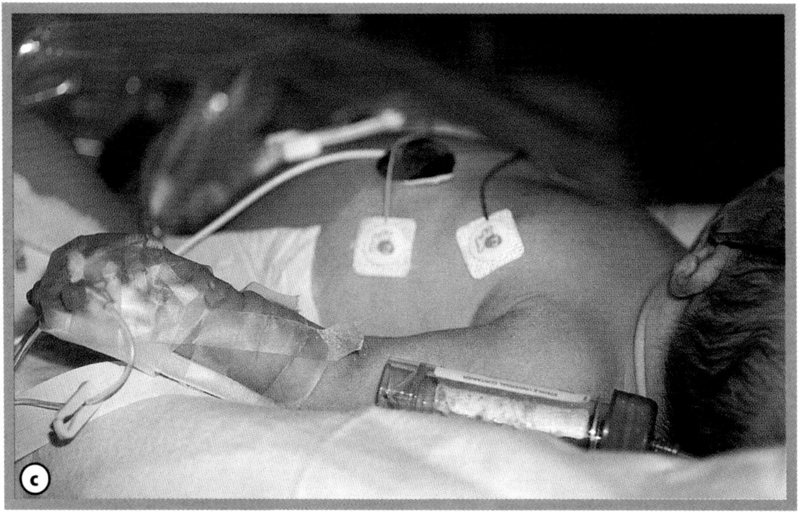

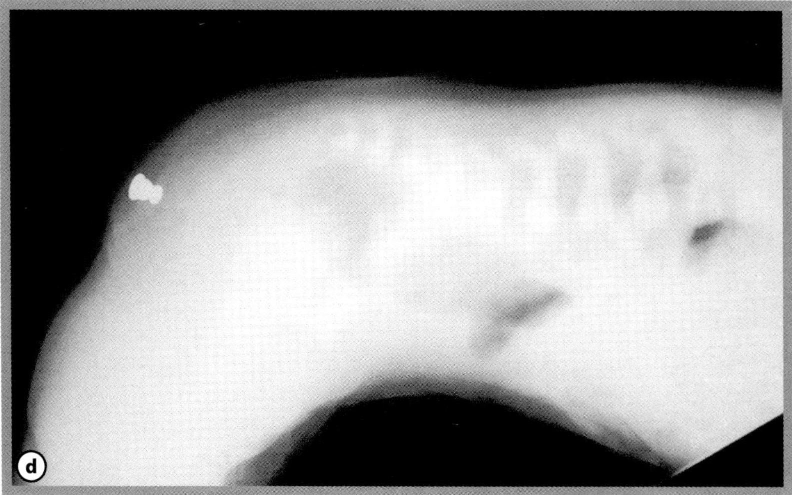

lateral radiograph showing absence of air in the rectum (**8.11d**). Mild forms of anal stenosis may just be associated with an anal web. Initial surgery requires a colostomy, and refashioning of the rectum and anal sphincters; anal opening requires multiple complex procedures over a number of years.

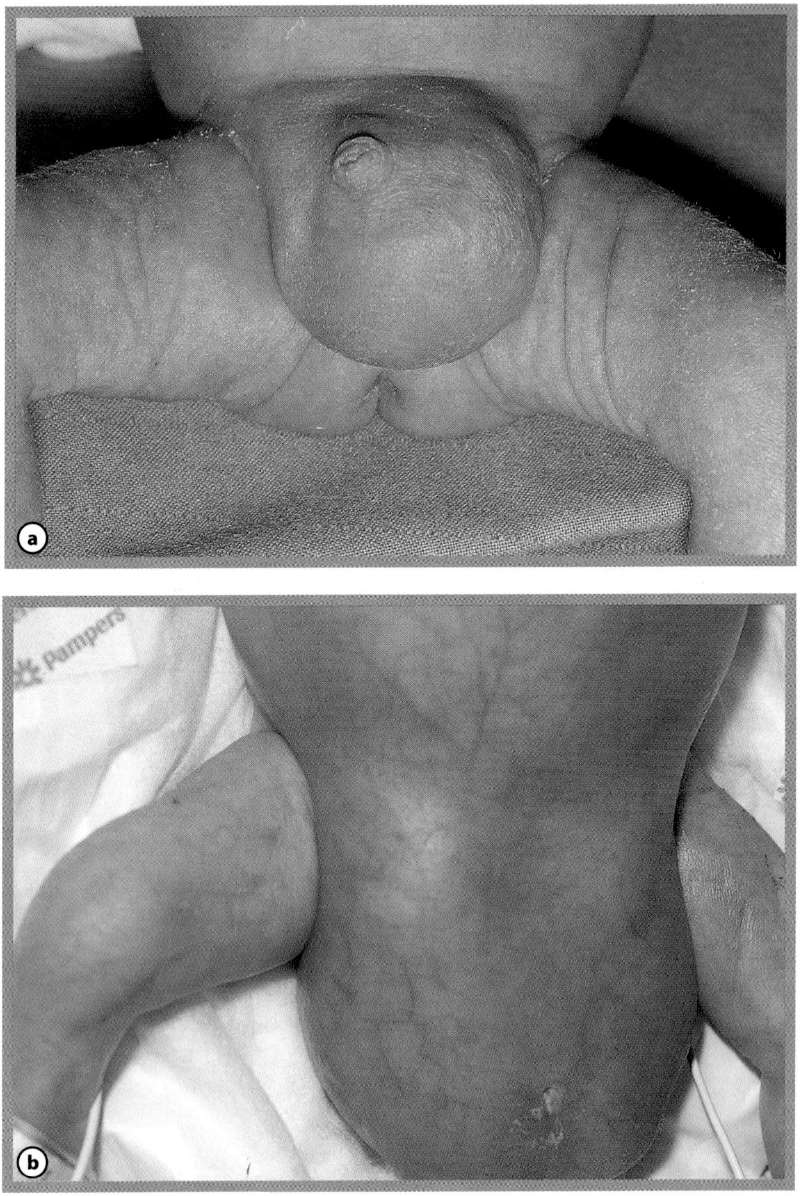

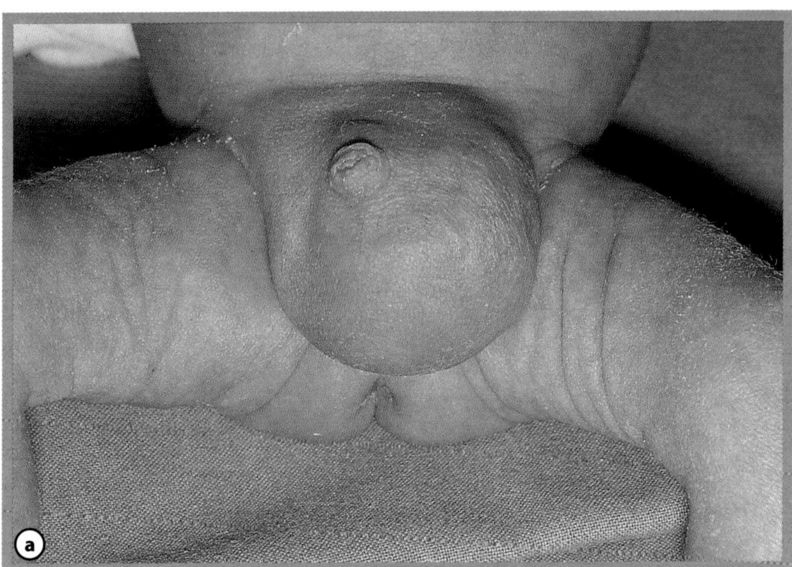

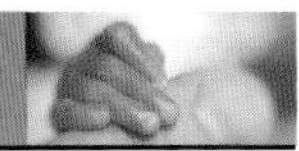

8.12a, 8.12b and 8.12c Bilateral inguinal hernia

Two infants are shown with inguino-scrotal hernias and, in the case of the second infant (**8.12b**), extensive herniation and obstruction of bowel has occurred (**8.12c**). The defect is caused by failure of obliteration of the patent processus vaginalis. Early elective surgical correction via inguinal herniotomy is advisable after diagnosis and, in the case of an acute presentation with an irreducible swelling, urgent surgery is required.

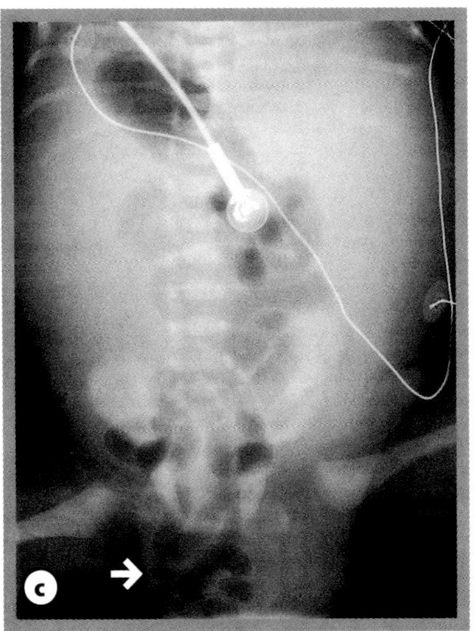

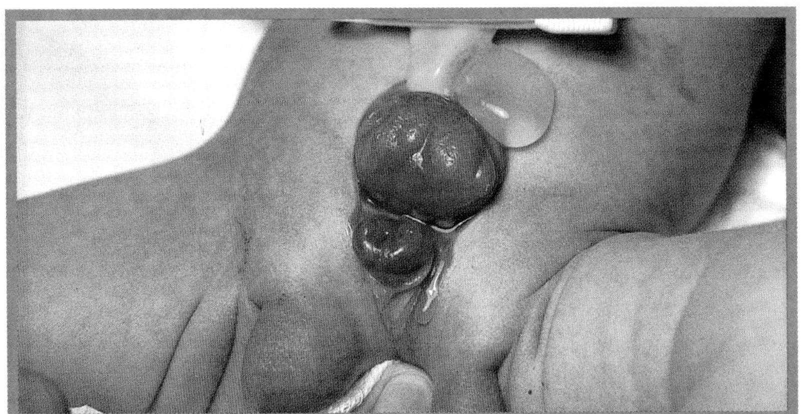

8.13 Bladder extrophy and epispadias

Bladder extrophy is seen with epispadias in this male infant. The umbilical cord arises from the superior border of the extrophy. The defect arises from a failure of mesodermal growth and a mid-line fusion of the endodermal and ectodermal layers. Reconstructive surgery is complex and an associated renal anomaly (e.g. vesico-ureteric reflux) is common.

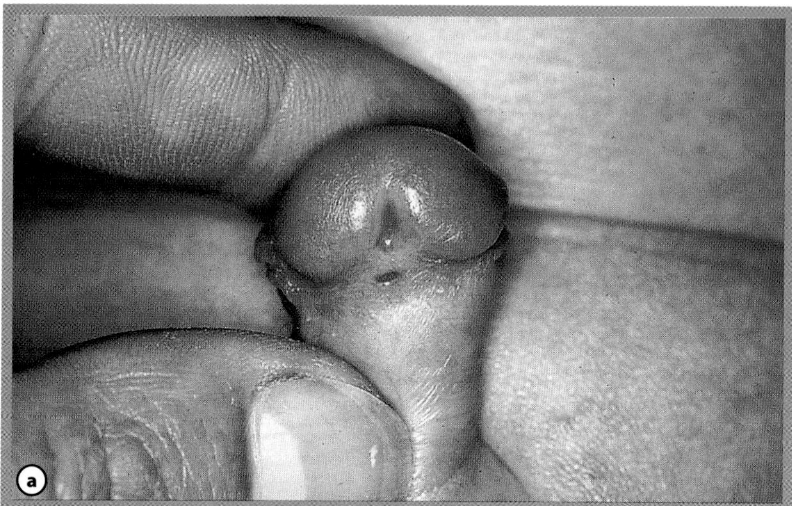

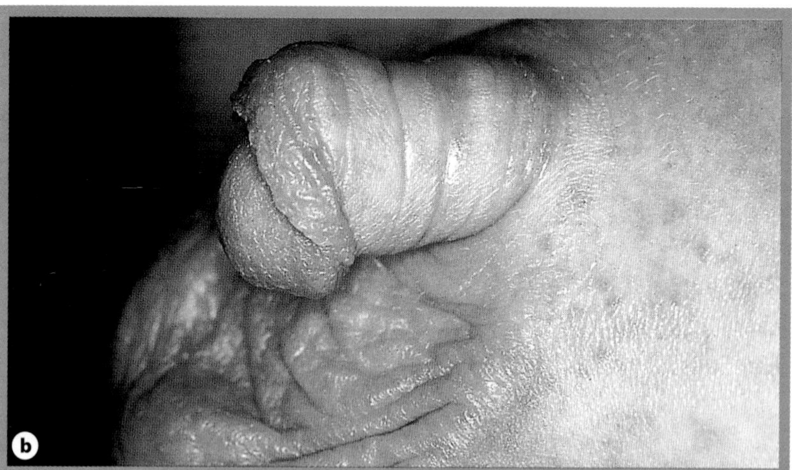

8.14a, 8.14b, 8.14c and 8.14d Hypospadias
This is a relatively frequent congenital abnormality occurring in about 1 out of 400 live male births. A mild defect is shown (**8.14a**) and also inferior displacement of the meatal opening within the glands and a hooded prepuce (**8.14b**). The more severe end of the spectrum (**8.14c**) is when the urethral

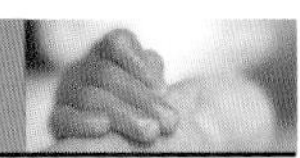

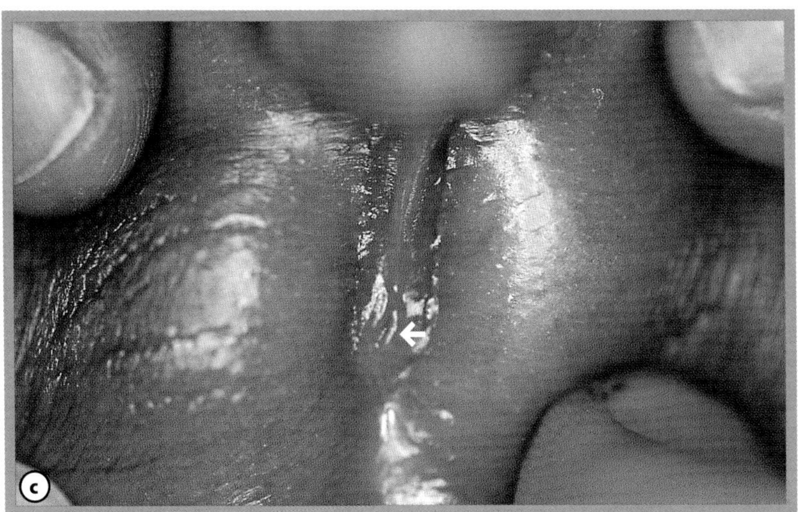

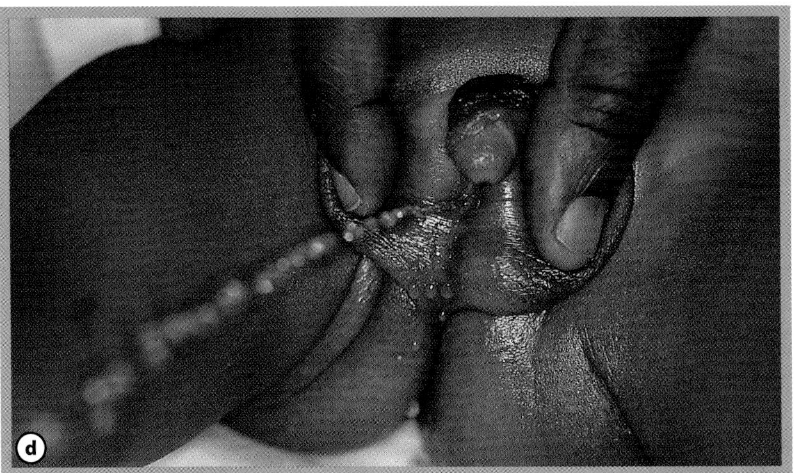

opening occurs within the scrotum: urination appears to come from 'within' the scrotum (**8.14d**). It is also possible for the urethral opening to be in the perineum. In addition to abnormal positioning of the meatus, there is usually a deficiency of the foreskin as well as the chordee, causing ventral flexion of the penile shaft.

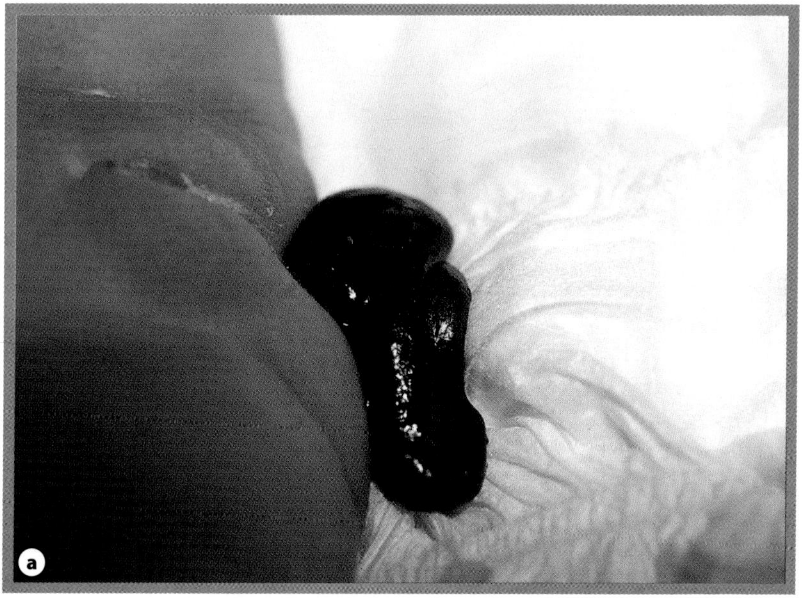

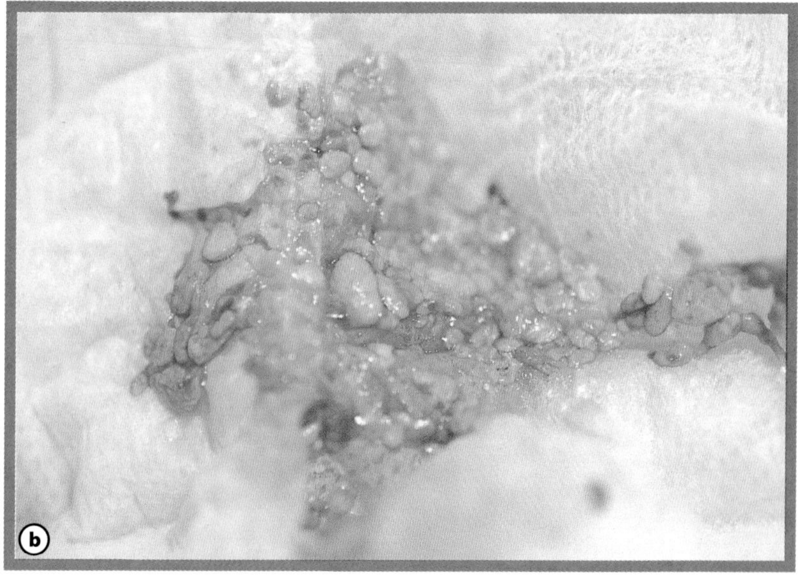

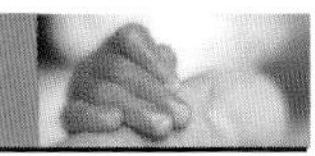

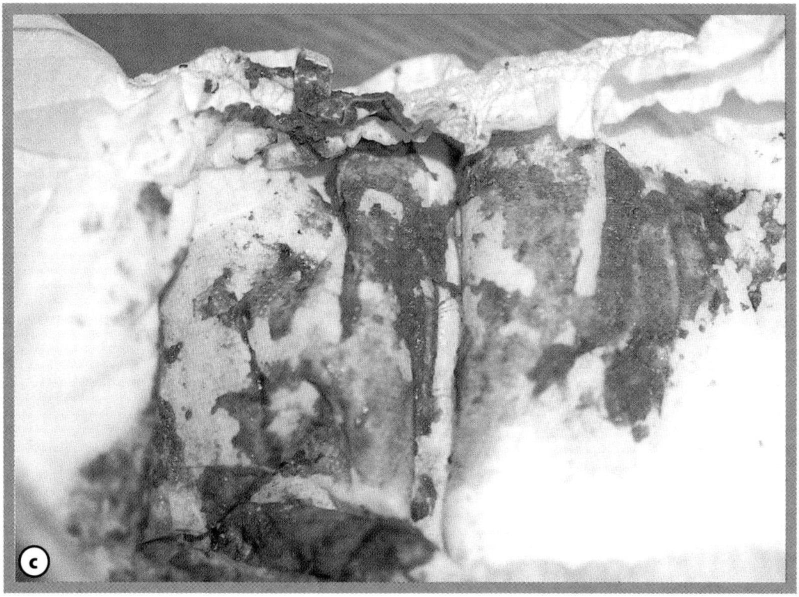

8.15a, 8.15b and 8.15c Different appearance of stools during infancy
The majority of infants pass meconium within the first 48 hours of birth (**8.15a**). Failure to do so needs to be further explored. Passage of meconium *in utero* is often a sign of foetal distress and can lead to meconium aspiration syndrome. Seedy yellow stools are usually found in breast-fed infants (**8.15b**). The stool is usually soft and not offensive. The frequency of opening the bowels is very variable. Some infants may open their bowels with each feed, others may go for days without opening their bowels. As long the infant is well and the stool is soft the parents can be reassured. Green stools are common and are often not associated with any underlying abnormality (**8.15c**).

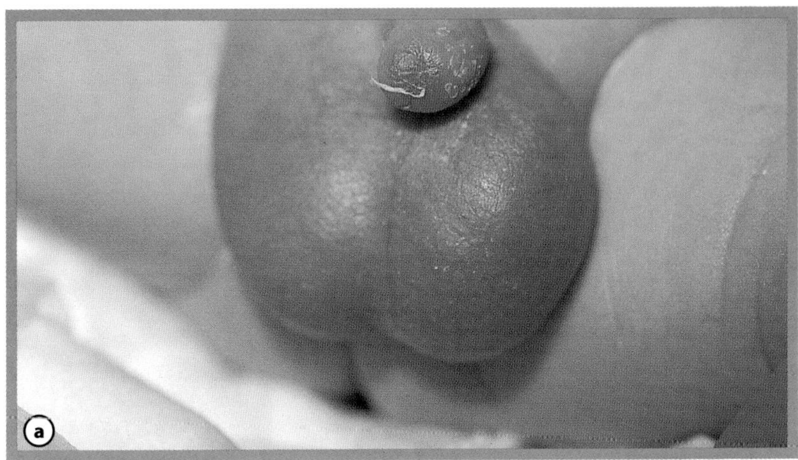

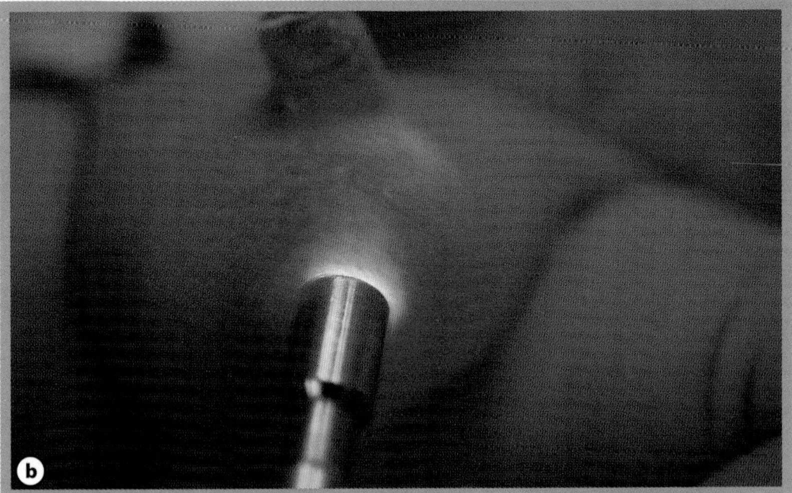

8.16a and 8.16b Bilateral hydrocoeles
These are caused by the persistence of isolated portions of the processus vaginalis, resulting in either hydrocoeles of the testes as shown or localized encysted hydrocoeles of the spermatic cord. Spontaneous resolution is common but surgery may be required if they persist, particularly beyond 12 months of age. A bright light source clearly transilluminates the hydrocele (**8.16b**).

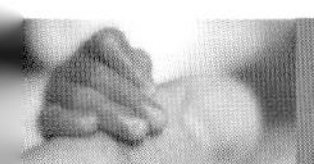

9 Skeletal

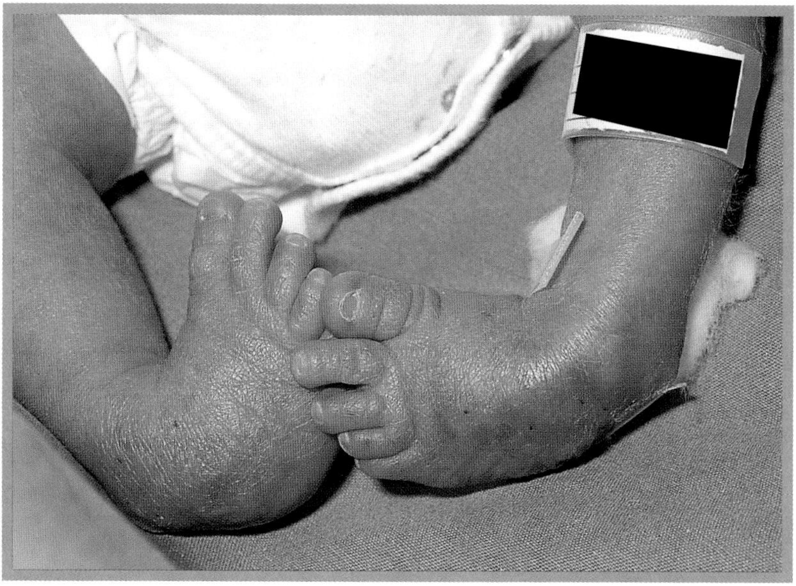

9.1 Bilateral talipes equinovarus

This deformity, club foot, may be either fixed or positional. The latter is more common as a result of intra-uterine posture and resolves usually with physiotherapy. The fixed deformity however is complex to treat and may be unilateral or bilateral. The defect may also be associated with neuromuscular disorders (e.g. spina bifida).

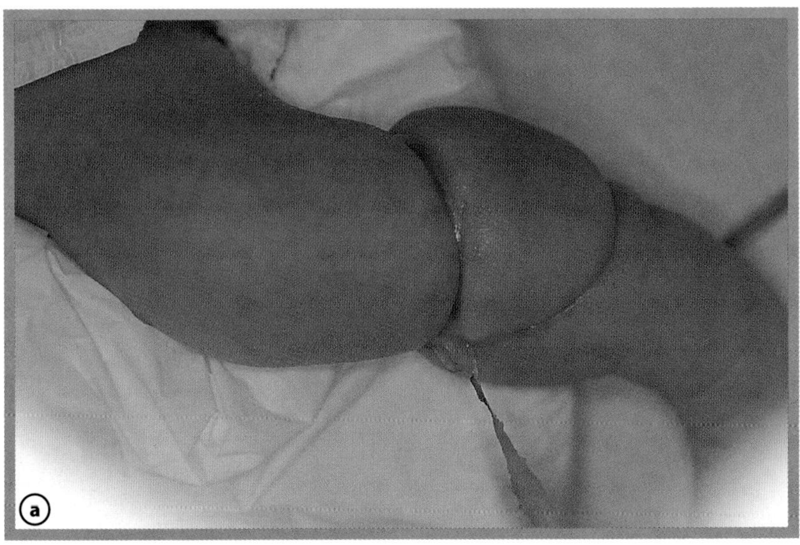

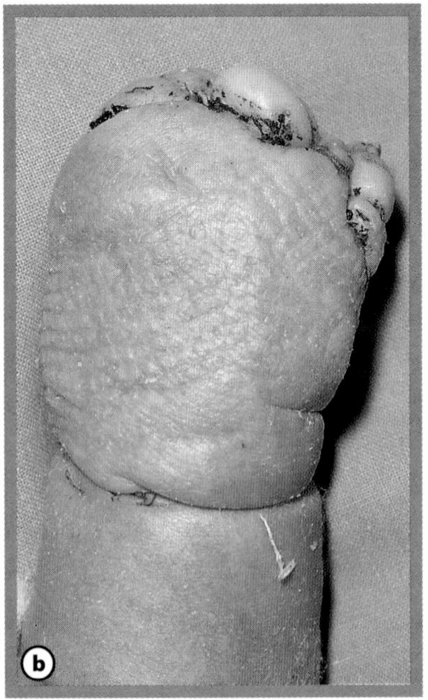

9.2a, 9.2b, 9.2c, 9.2d and 9.2e Amniotic bands

The restriction deformities shown include complete amputation of the fingers, deep constriction bands around the lower limb and a band around the thorax. These injuries are thought to be caused by free-floating amniotic bands, although the mechanism is disputed. However, the presence of these bands is clearly shown in **9.2a**. Furthermore, an amniotic band is shown *in situ* (**9.2d**). The defect may involve all of the tissues down as far as bone and (**9.2e**) shows a resultant congenital fracture of the distal radius and ulna. In severe cases extensive reconstructive surgery is required.

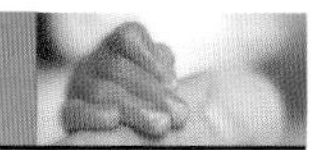

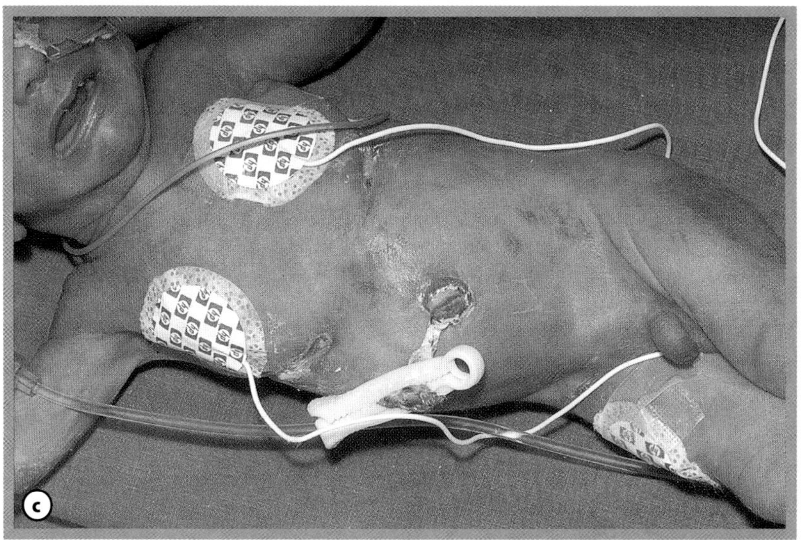

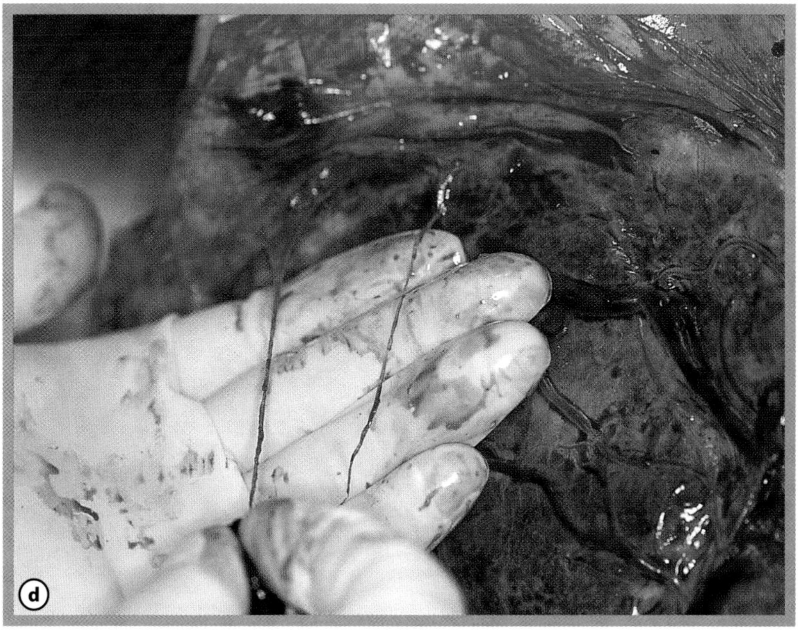

d

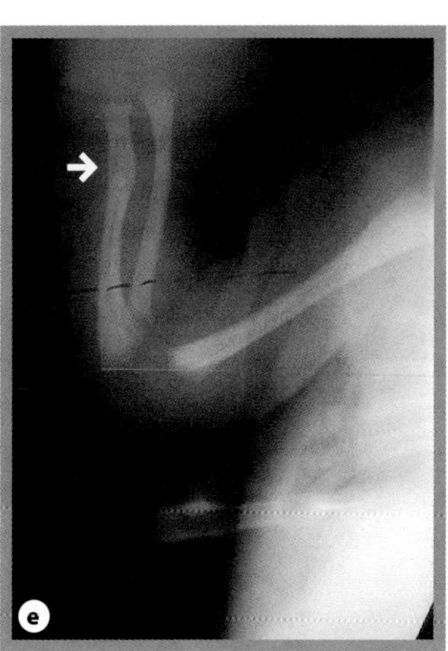

9.2 Amniotic bands continued

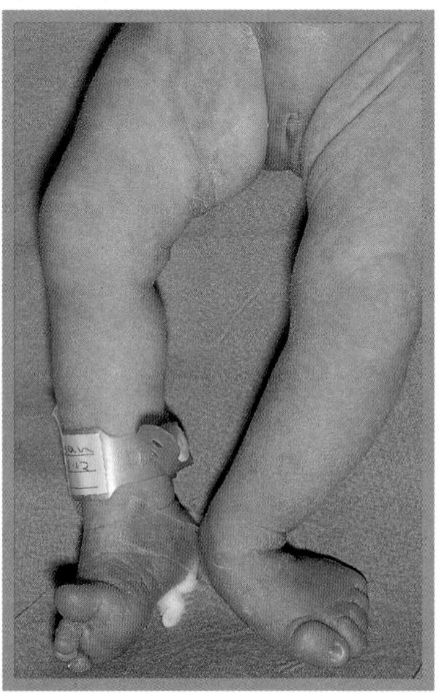

9.3 Bilateral talipes calcaneovalgus

This common finding is most likely caused by intra-uterine positioning. Dorsiflexion is excessive and plantar flexion is reduced. The condition resolves spontaneously in the vast majority of patients and treatment consists of physiotherapy with stretching exercises to bring the foot back to the neutral position.

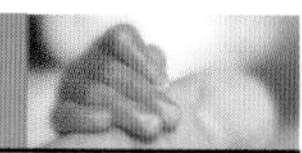

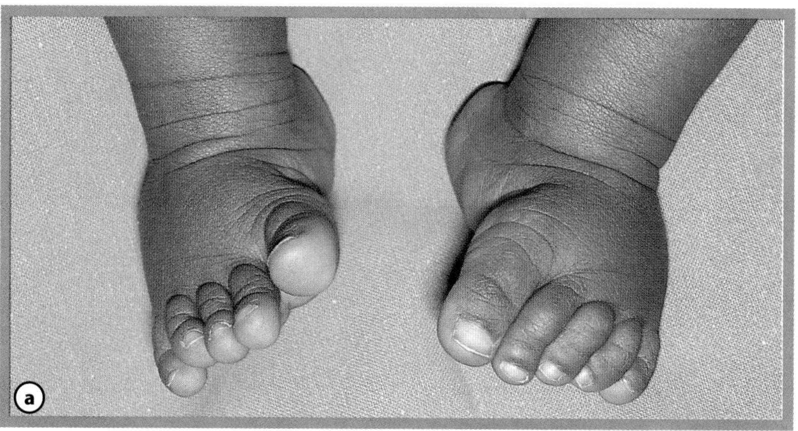

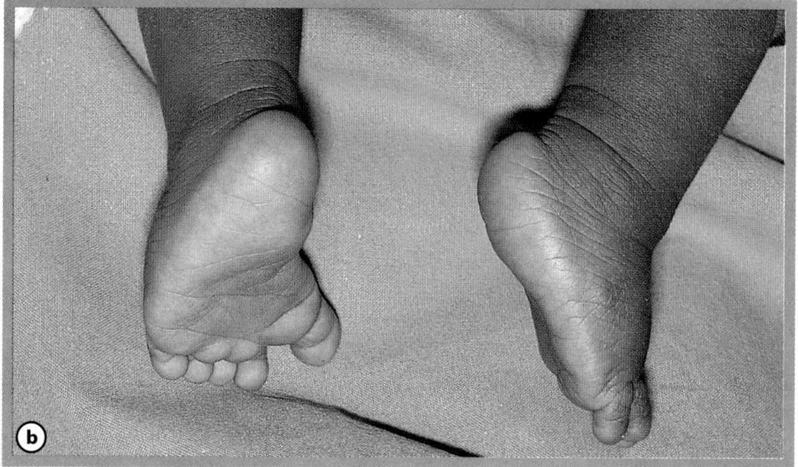

9.4a and 9.4b Metatarsus adductus varus

This condition is defined as an internal angulation of the forefoot or metatarsals on a neutral and flexible hindfoot. It is thought to result from intra-uterine positioning. There is a possible increased incidence of congenital hip dislocations found associated with the condition, however, spontaneous correction usually occurs. In severe cases where the forefoot cannot be brought to neutral alignment with the hindfoot with passive manipulation, a short course of casting may be needed.

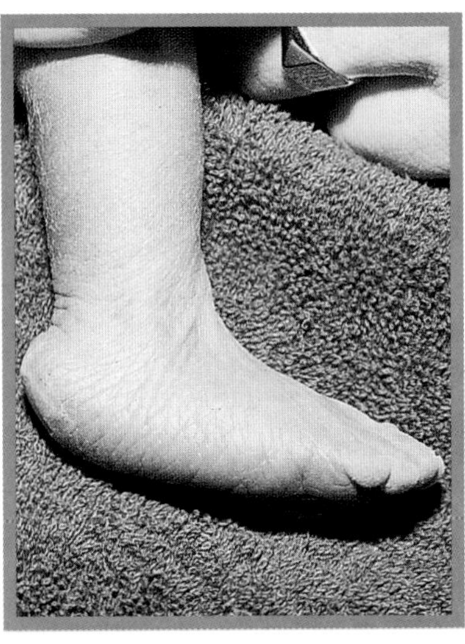

9.5 Rocker bottom feet

This is a rare finding and in the majority of patients is associated with an underlying abnormality, particularly those involving the central nervous system such as myelodysplasia and sacral agenesis. It is also seen in Turner syndrome and Edward syndrome as well as arthrogryposis.

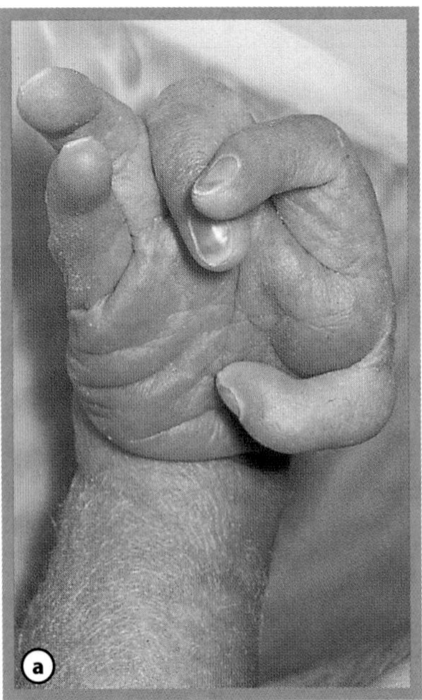

9.6a, 9.6b and 9.6c Skeletal dysplasia

This child exhibits abnormalities of the hands, feet and spine and is classified as a skeletal dysplasia. This term embraces a variety of clinical complexes including spondylo-epiphyseal dysplasia, multiple epiphyseal dysplasia and pseudo-achondroplasia. Skeletal dysplasia may be part of a syndrome with other abnormalities (e.g. short stature in Down syndrome and Turner syndrome).

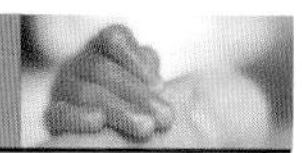

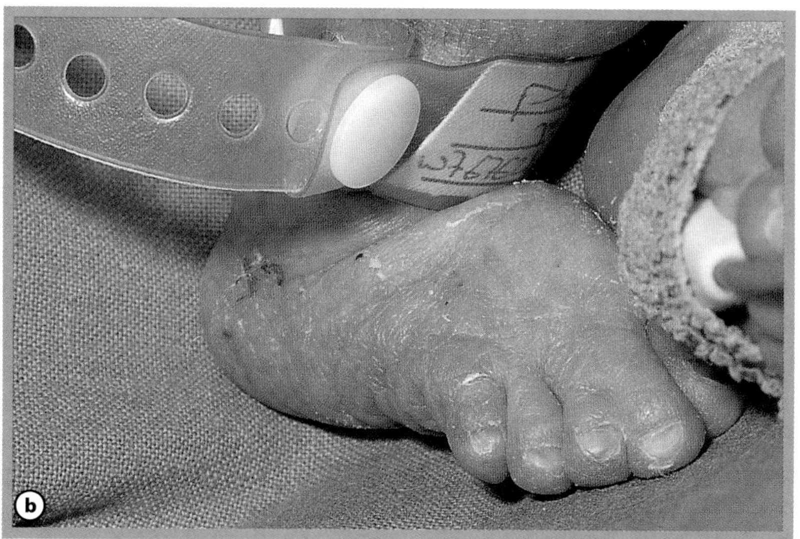

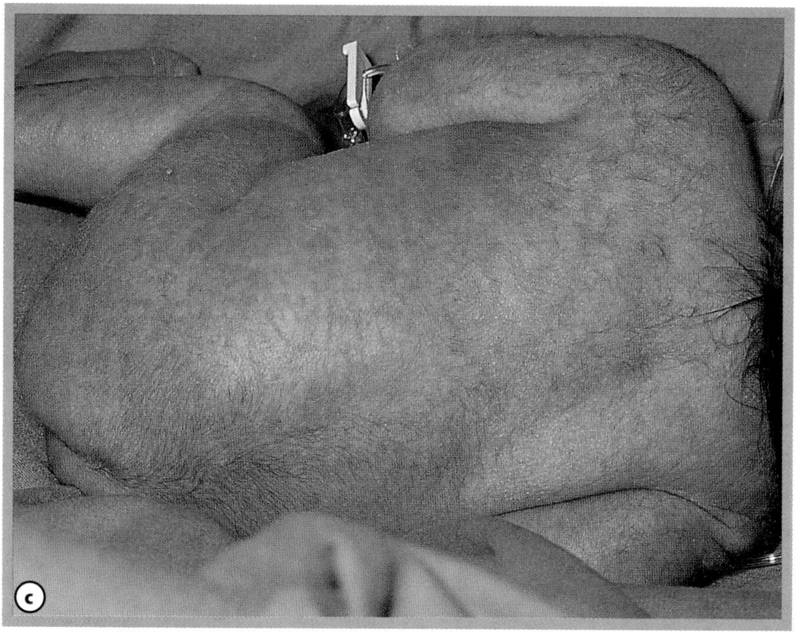

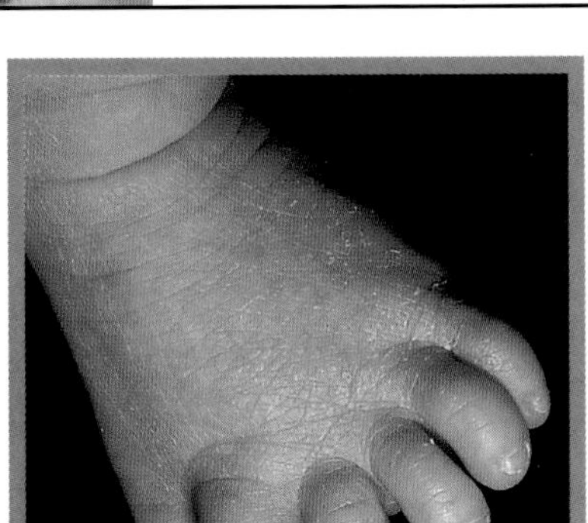

9.7 Polydactyly

Excess digits may occur in isolation or in association with a range of congenital disorders, for example, Carpenter syndrome (craniosynostosis, congenital heart disease and learning disability). The extra digit may have no bony attachment and be considered simply as a skin tag or it may be a true functioning digit. Surgical excision is required and early referral to a plastic surgeon is warranted.

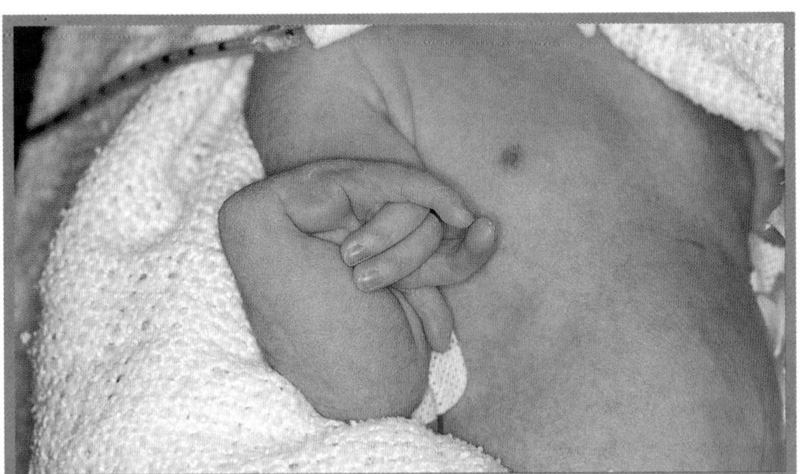

9.8 Club hand

Club hand is due to congenital absence of the radius, resulting in the curved, internally rotated ulna as shown. In this patient, as in the majority, the finding was associated with other major anomalies, in particular, oesophageal atresia, tracheo-oesophageal fistula and renal abnormalities, the VATER complex. An absence of the radius also occurs as part of the TAR syndrome with thrombocytopenia.

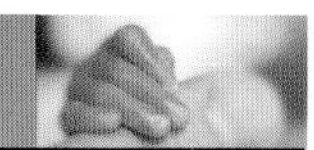

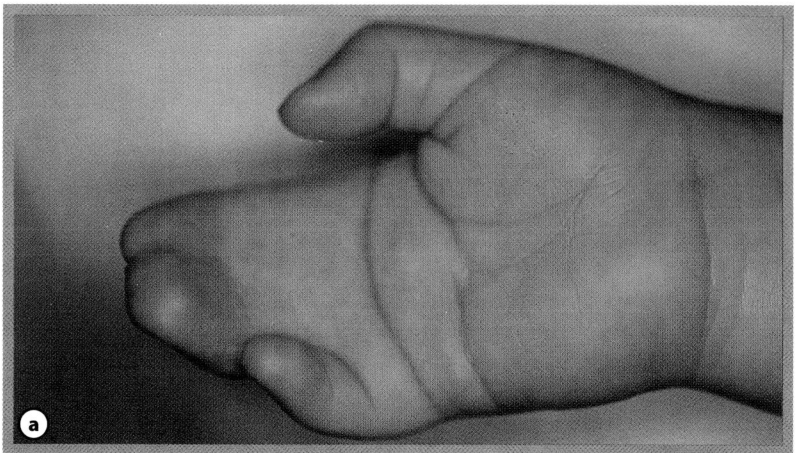

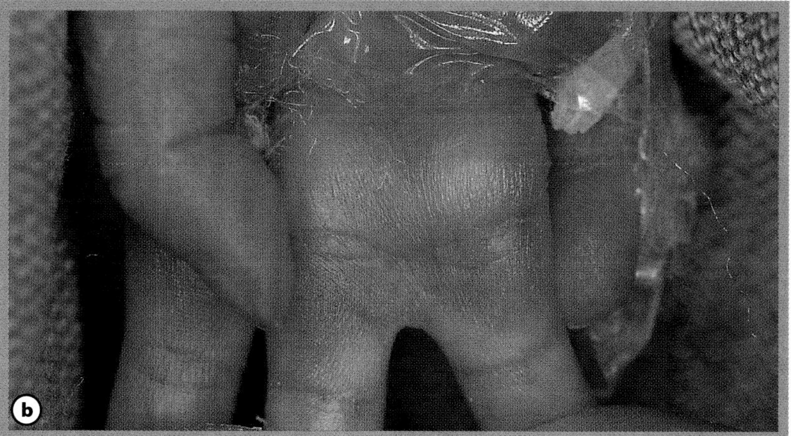

9.9a and 9.9b Syndactyly
Two different patients are shown, with bony attachment (**9.9a**) and without (**9.9b**). The former requires major reconstructive hand surgery to achieve independently functioning digits. Syndactyly may occur as an isolated finding, although commonly forms part of the clinical expression of a wide range of disorders, for example, Apert syndrome (craniosynostosis, mid-facial hypoplasia, learning disability).

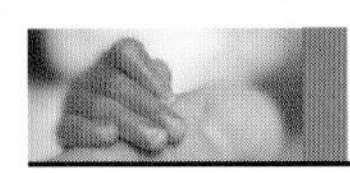

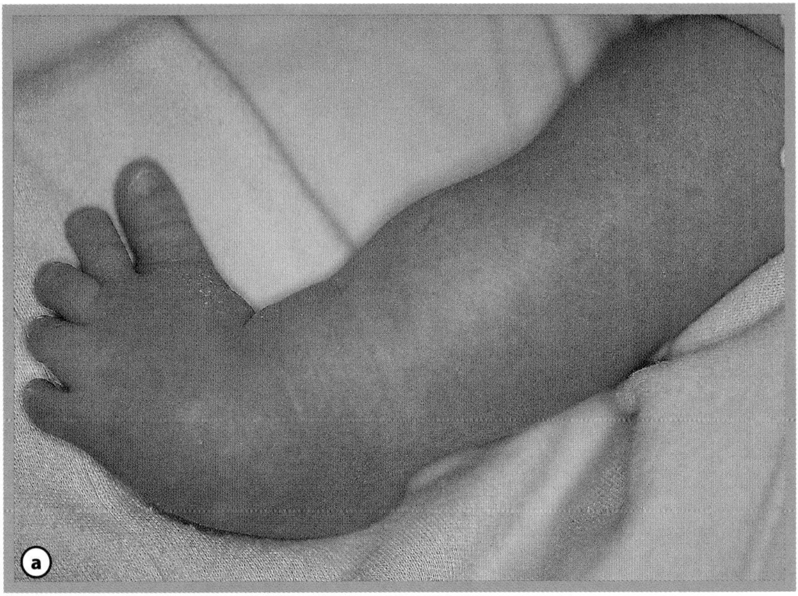

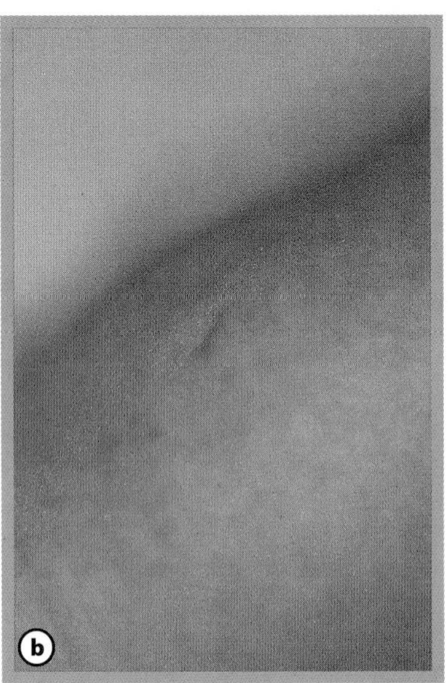

9.10a and 9.10b Camptomelic dysplasia

This infant showed the classical features of this autosomal recessive condition with short, bowed lower limbs with a dimple on the anterior aspect of the tibia. Associated features include a low nasal bridge, micrognathia and a small thorax. Although this infant was a phenotypic female, the chromosomes were XY. The usual outcome is death in early infancy due to respiratory insufficiency. This patient, however, has survived well beyond this period.

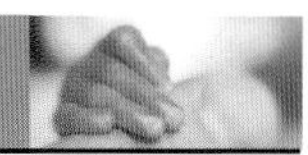

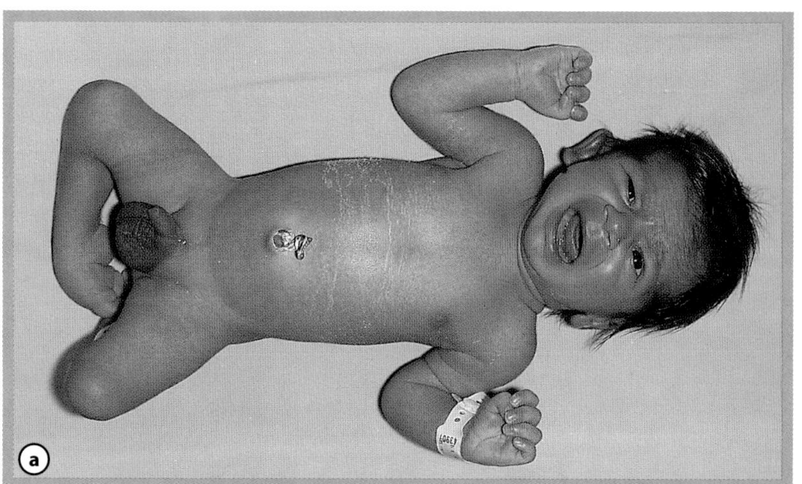

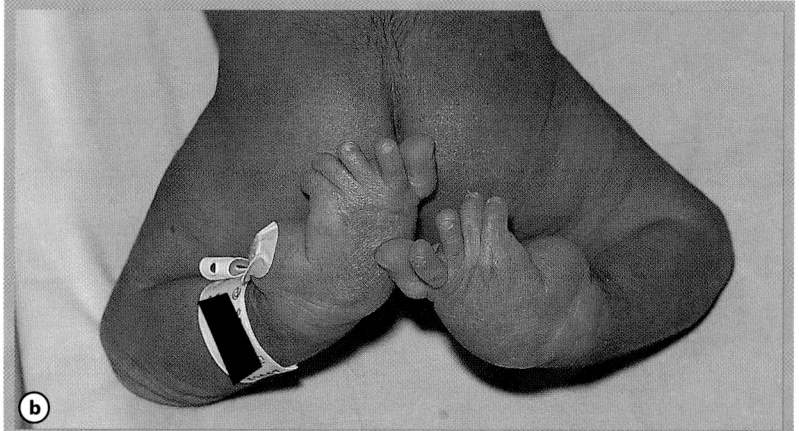

9.11a and 9.11b Arthrogryposis

This clinical complex may be caused by a variety of disorders, all of which have as their common pathway intra-uterine restriction of joint movement. This may be caused by either oligohydramnios or by factors severely reducing muscle tone and hence mobility in the foetus. Treatment consists of correcting the deformity as well as addressing the often severe muscle weakness. Cognitive function is not usually affected.

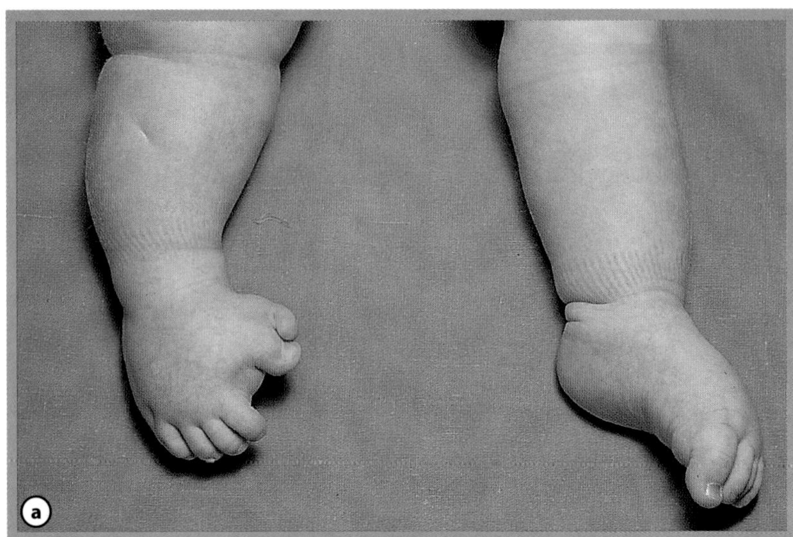

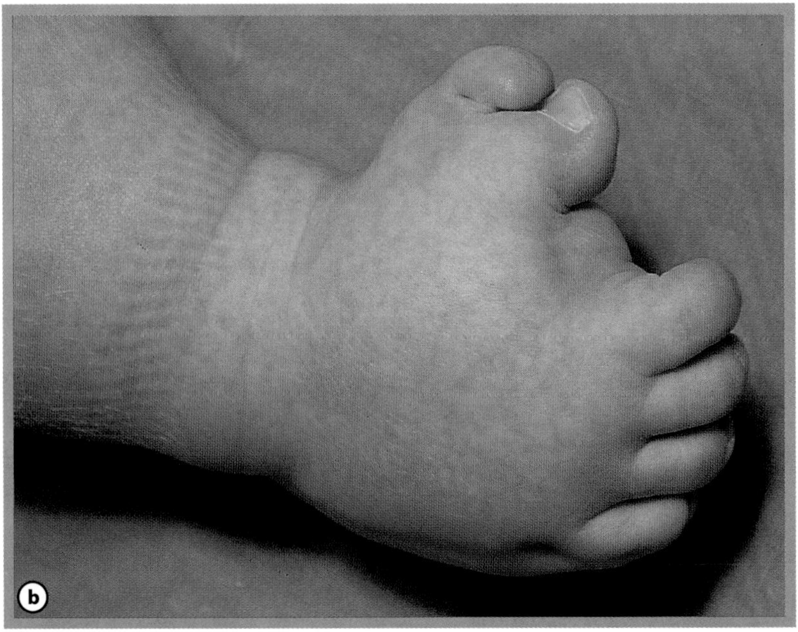

b

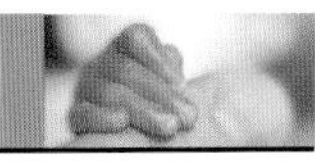

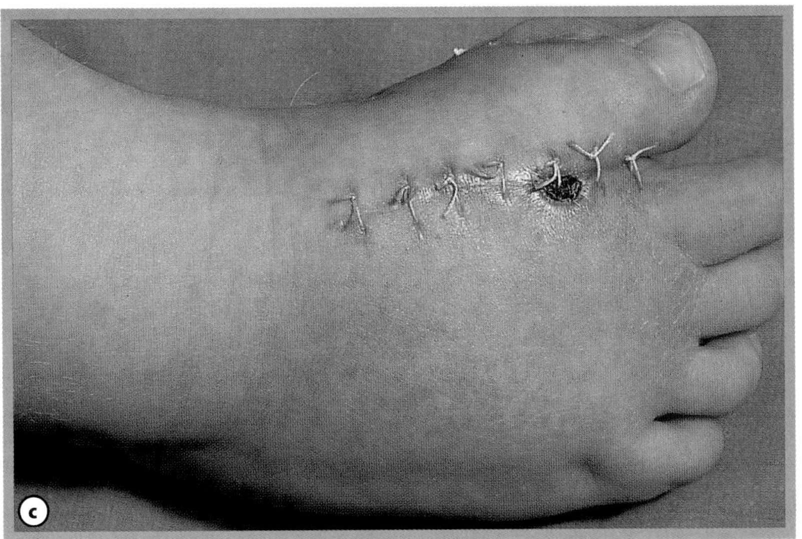

9.12a, 9.12b and 9.12c Split hand and foot syndrome
Central ray defects of the hand and foot are developmental defects that result in deletion to various degrees of the central rays of the hands and feet. The phenotypic expression of this syndrome may vary from complete absence of all elements of the hand and foot to various other manifestations with less severe deficiencies. The final picture (**9.12c**) shows a good cosmetic and functional outcome after surgery.

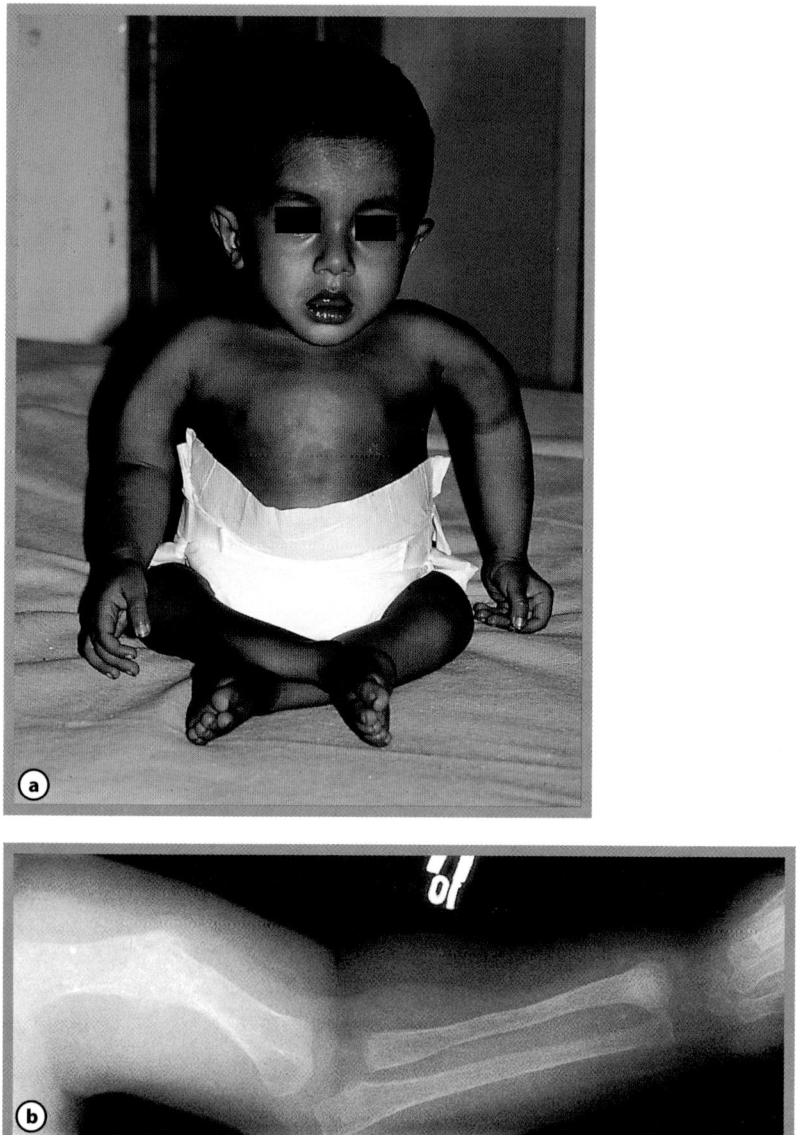

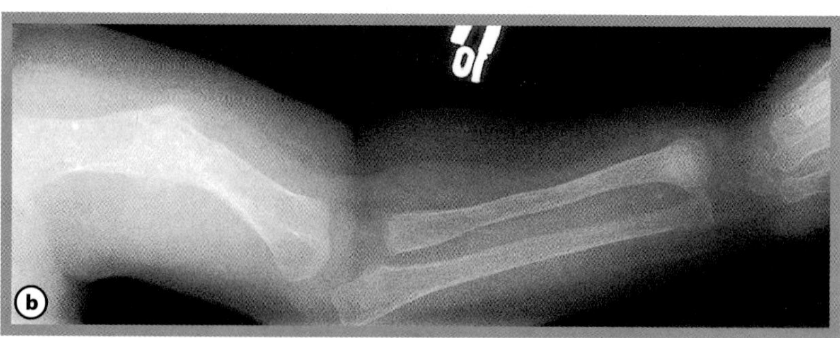

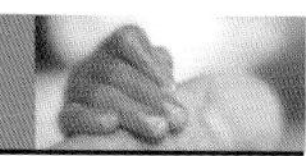

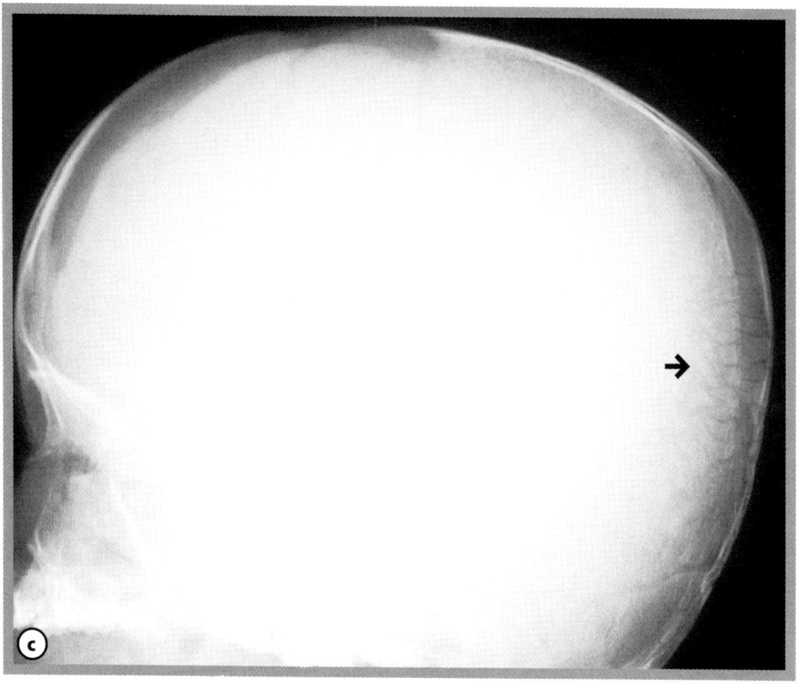

9.13a, 9.13b and 9.13c Osteogenesis imperfecta

This patient has osteogenesis imperfecta type III (autosomal recessive) which is characterized by fractures in the newborn period with progressively more severe disease due to multiple fractures. Death is likely by the fourth decade due to cardiorespiratory insufficiency. The sclera is only blue for a short period in infancy and then gradually changes to a normal colour. An x-ray on day 1 (**9.13b**) shows a congenital fracture of the humerus as well as the distal radius with callus formation. The final picture (**9.13c**) shows the presence of wormian bones.

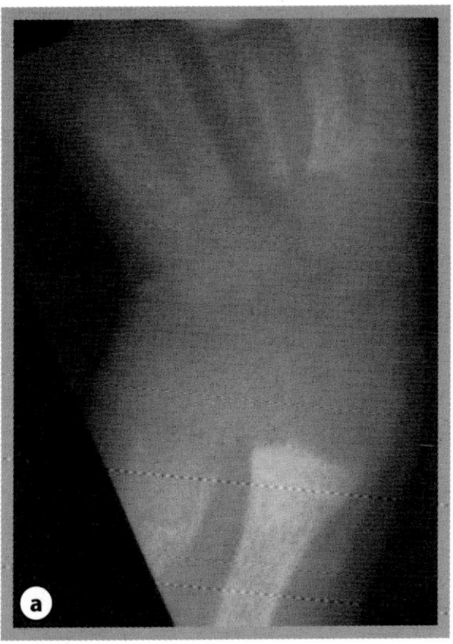

9.14a, 9.14b and 9.14c Rickets

This infant's wrist radiograph (**9.14a**) displays the classical features of rickets with frayed radial and ulnar metaphyses with slight expansion. The radiological features are often evident, as in this case, before the appearance of clinical signs. The centre picture (**9.14b**) shows bilateral fractured femurs associated with severe rickets. The final picture (**9.14c**) shows classical bowed legs. Neonatal rickets is commonly caused by hypophosphataemia and treatment consists of phosphate supplementation in the first instance followed by addition of 1-alpha calcidol if required.

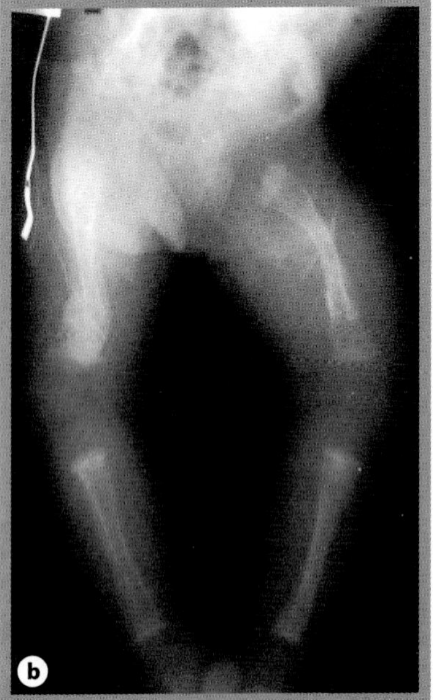

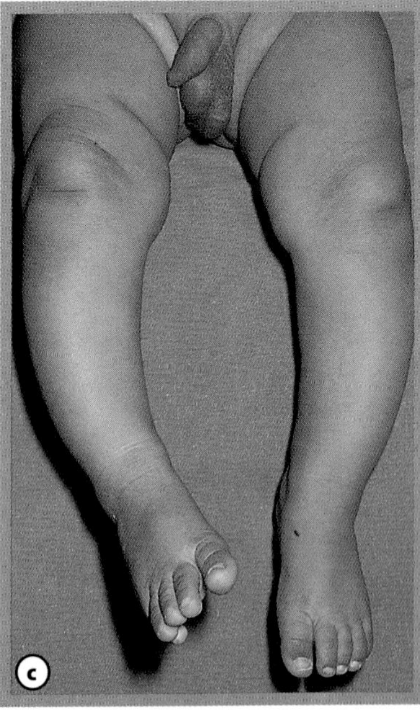

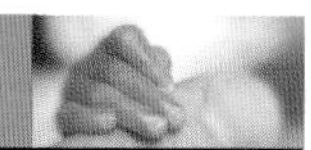

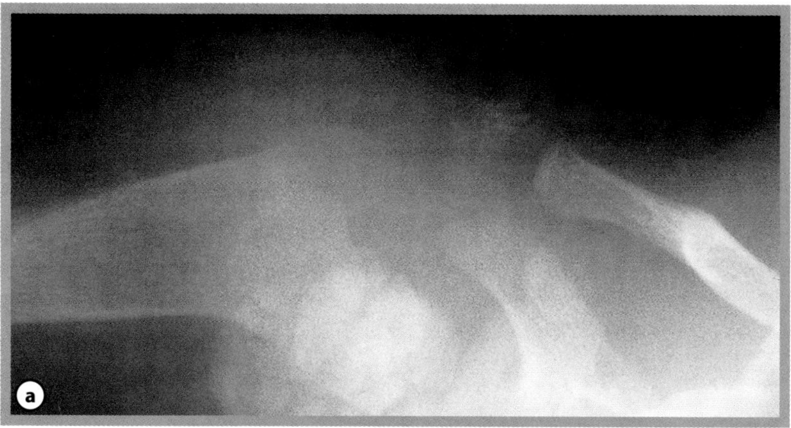

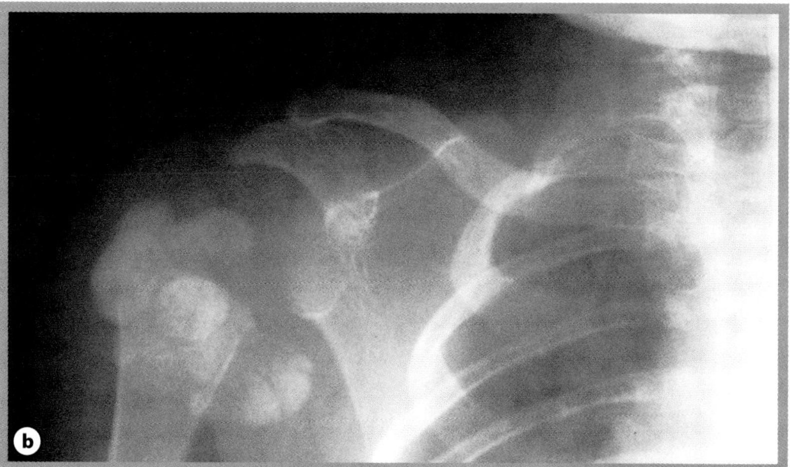

9.15a and 9.15b Tumoral calcinosis

This infant was born at 28-weeks gestation and was ventilated for 4 days. He had a chest drain inserted on the right side. A routine follow-up film showed calcification around the head of the humerus. Tumoral calcinosis is a benign condition of unknown aetiology. Trauma is thought to be a possible precipitant. There is no associated calcification in other tissues and no biochemical abnormalities are noted. Spontaneous resolution may occur but surgery to remove the encapsulated calcified swelling is sometimes required.

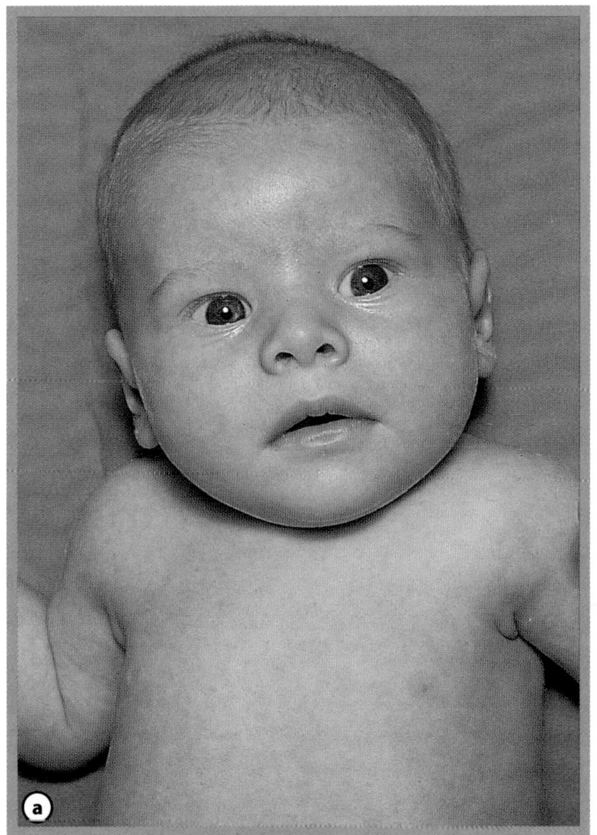

9.16a, 9.16b and 9.16c Sprengel's deformity
Bilateral Sprengel's shoulder is shown which is caused by failure of descent of the scapula. Unilateral deformity is more common but in this infant the defect was bilateral and indeed was initially confused with webbing of the neck. The chest radiograph shows high riding scapulae (**9.16c**). A magnetic resonance imaging scan of the neck and detailed views of the cervical spine showed no evidence of any other bony abnormality. Physiotherapy is the initial treatment of choice with corrective surgery later for cosmetic reasons.

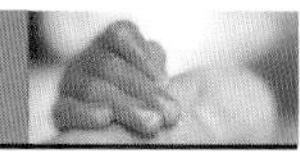

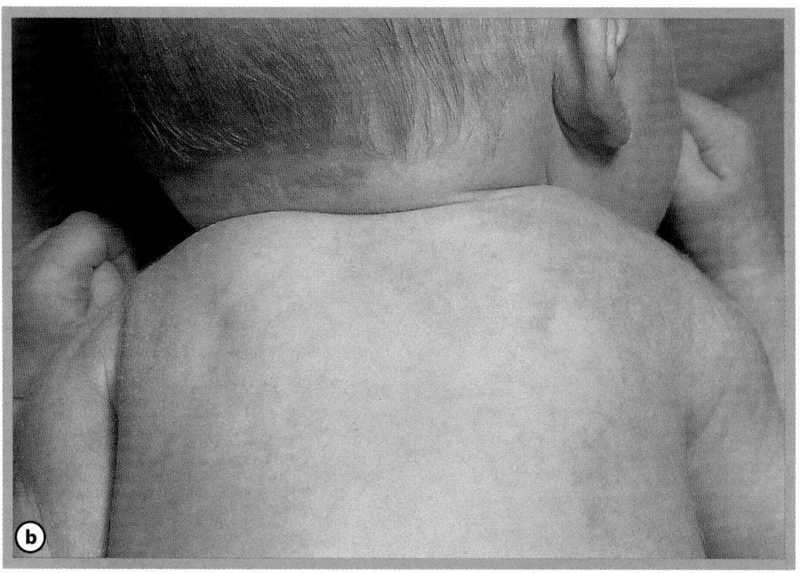

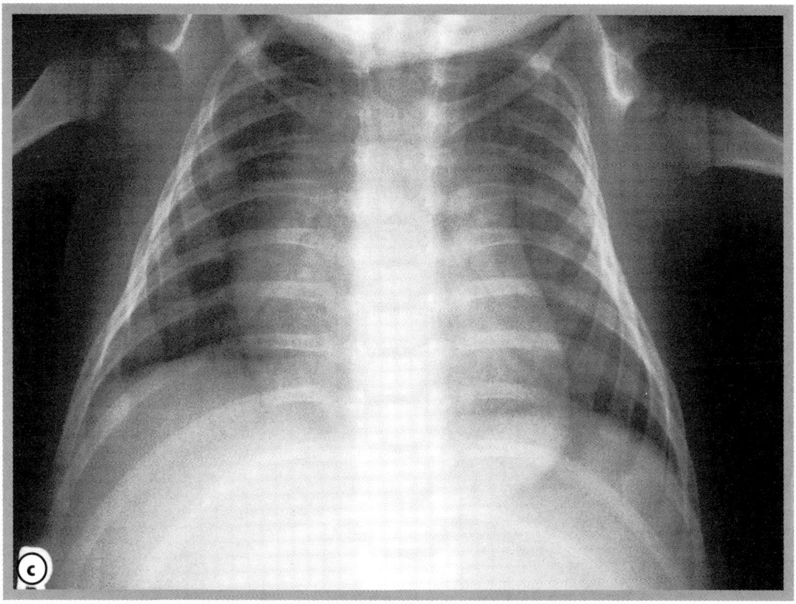

b

c

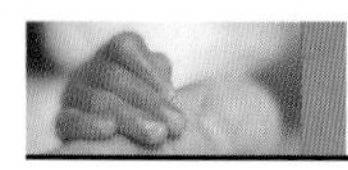

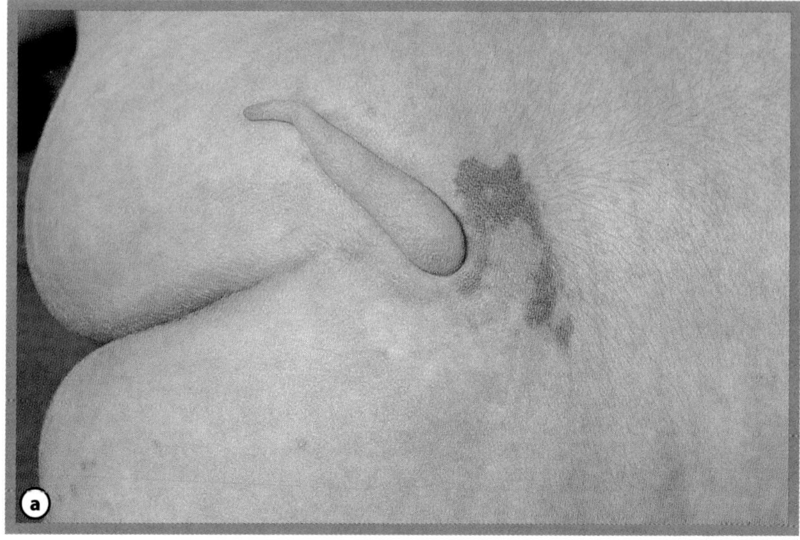

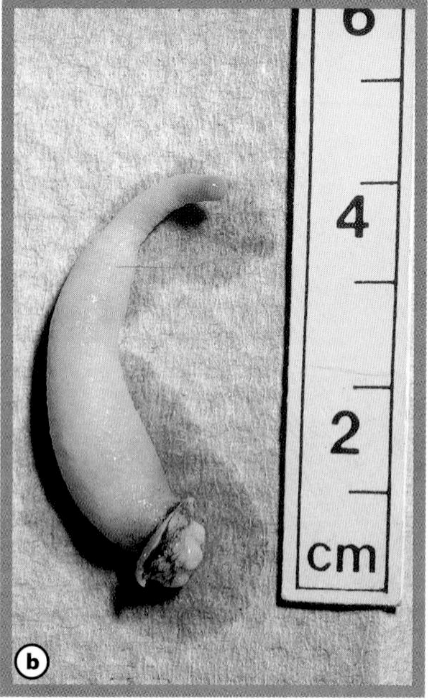

9.17a and 9.17b Congenital tail
This infant had a bony tail arising from its sacrum. This condition is exceptionally rare and there are only three recorded patients in the world.

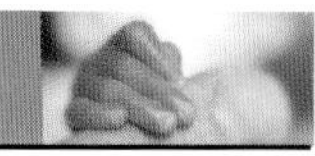

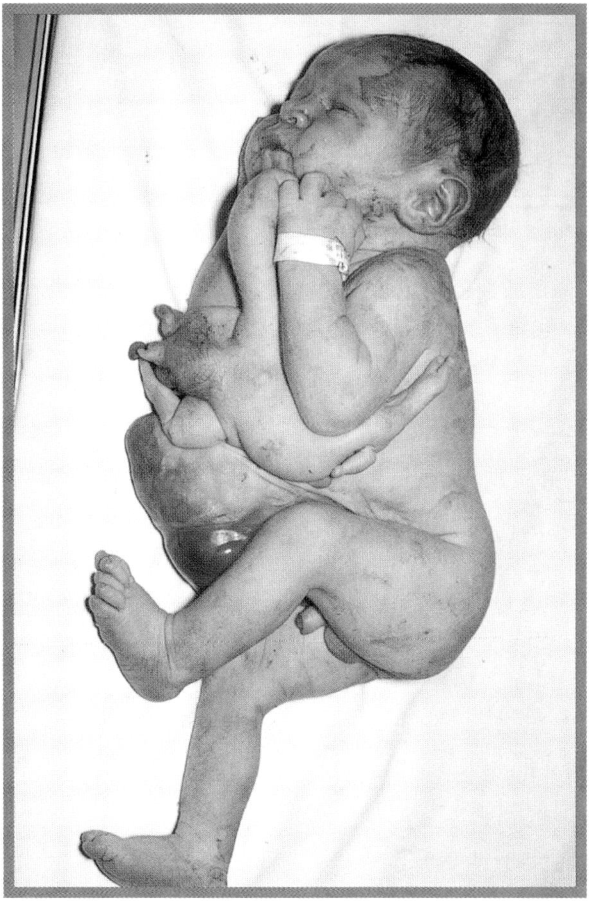

9.18 Siamese twin

This slide shows the remnants of a Siamese twin attached at the thorax to a fully formed male infant. Resection of the unviable twin was successful.

10 Syndromes

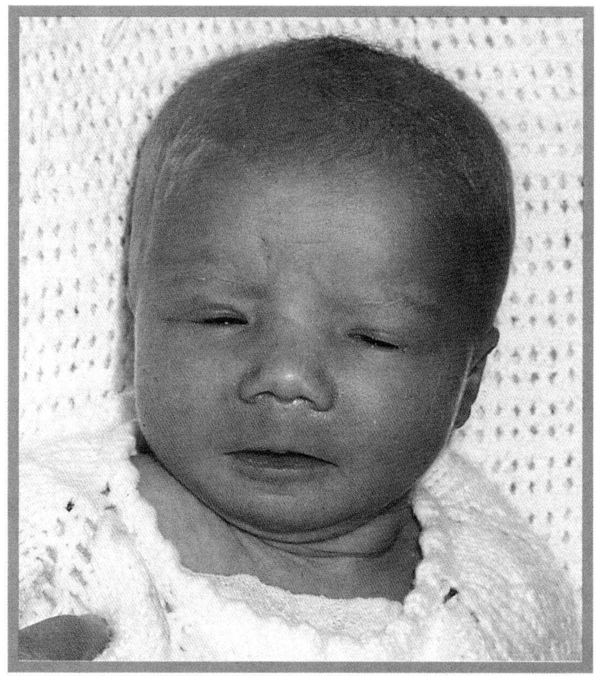

10.1 Fetal alcohol syndrome
The mother of this infant consumed 70 g of alcohol on a daily basis throughout pregnancy. The typical features of this syndrome include mild to moderate microcephaly, mid-facial hypoplasia, short palpebral fissures, thin upper lip, hirsutism in newborn period, shallow philtrum, epicanthic folds and mild ptosis. Learning difficulties are often present and can be severe.

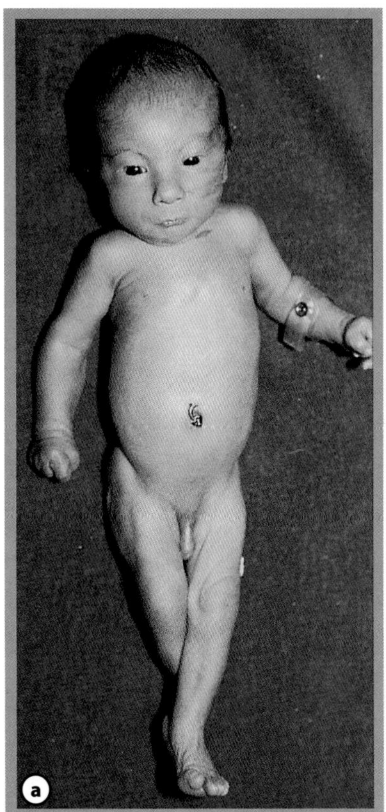

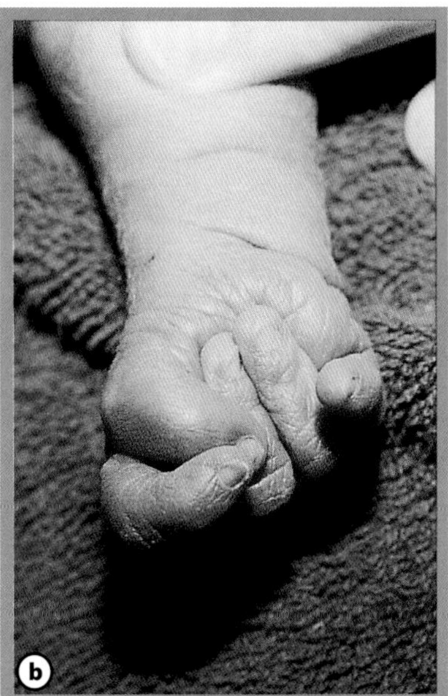

10.2a and 10.2b Trisomy 18 (Edward syndrome)
Edward syndrome has an incidence of 1 out of 5000. The classical features include a prominent occiput, a disproportionate long head and a small chin. The ears are low set and malformed (**10.2a**). The hands characteristically feature overlapping fingers e.g. second overlapping the third and occasionally, as shown here, fifth overlapping the fourth (**10.2b**). The majority of patients have a cardiac defect. Mental retardation in the 10% of patients that survive is severe.

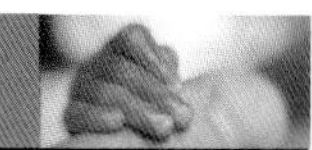

10.3a and 10.3b Down syndrome
This is the most common chromosomal anomaly and is present in 1 out of 600–700 live births. In most infants the abnormality is due to an extra chromosome 21. Diagnosis is based on the characteristic findings of upward slanting eyes, prominent epicanthic folds, flat nasal bridge, protruding tongue, short neck, flat occiput and hypotonia. A single transverse palmar crease and a sandal gap between the first and second toe, as shown in **10.3b**, are typical. Congenital heart disease, as seen in this infant who is cyanosed, is present in 40%. This infant also had duodenal atresia.

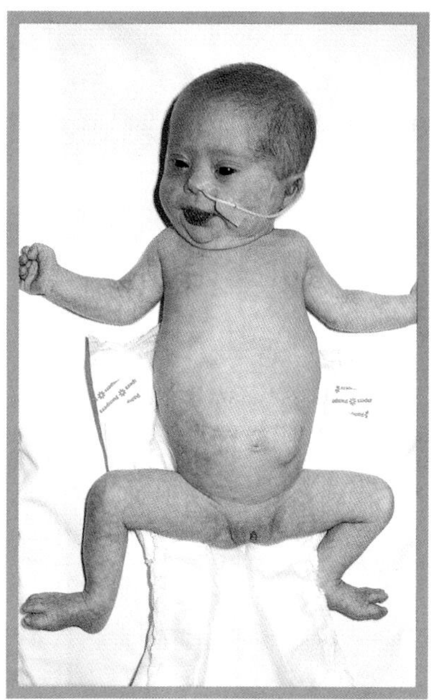

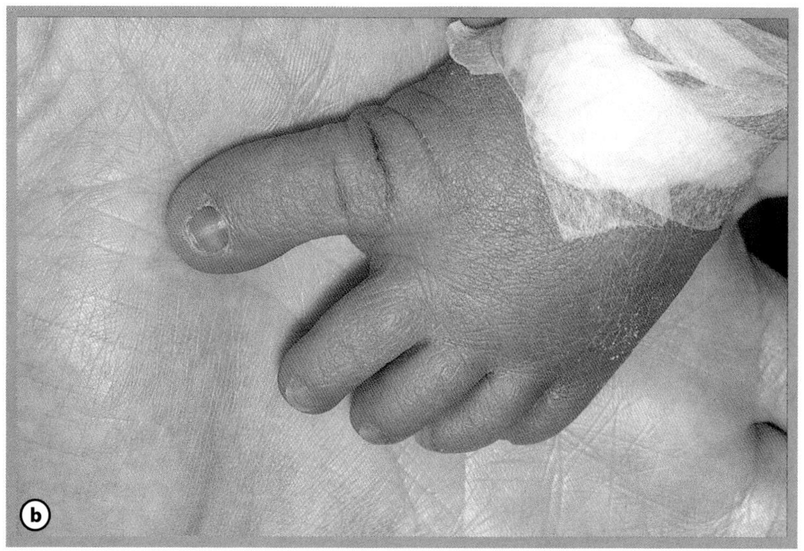

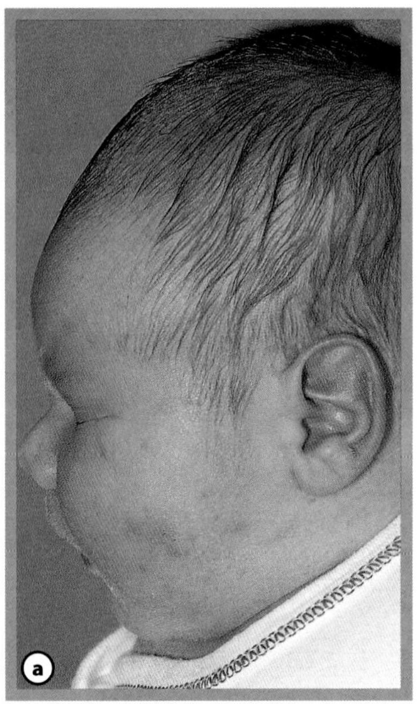

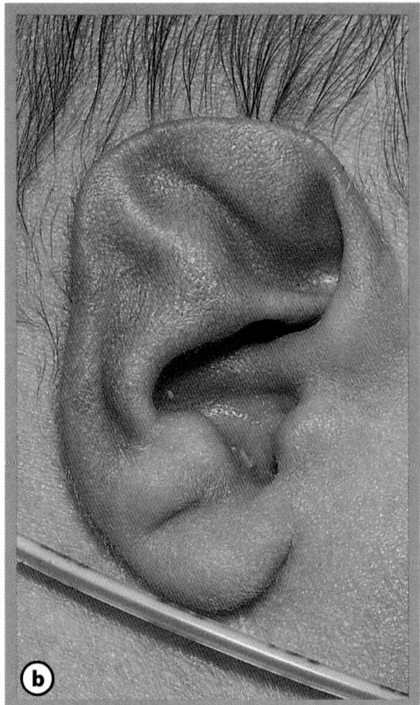

10.4a and 10.4b Beckwith–Wiedemann syndrome
This infant shows the classical vertical ear creases of this syndrome which is also associated with profound neonatal hypoglycaemia. Other features that may be present include increased birth weight, a large tongue, coarse facies, organomegaly, exomphalos and a predisposition to Wilm's tumour. It is linked to chromosome 11p15.5.

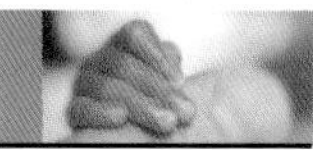

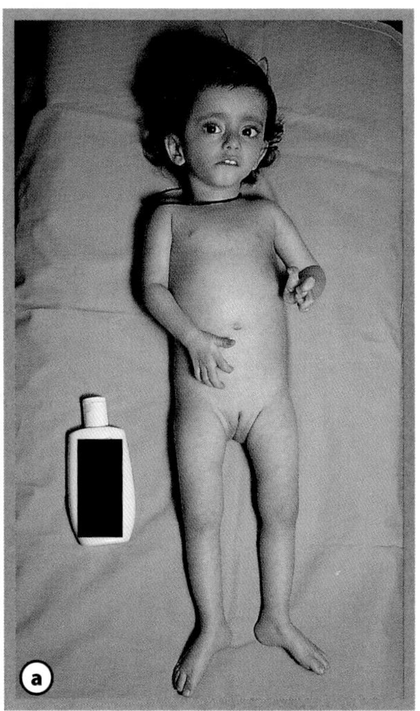

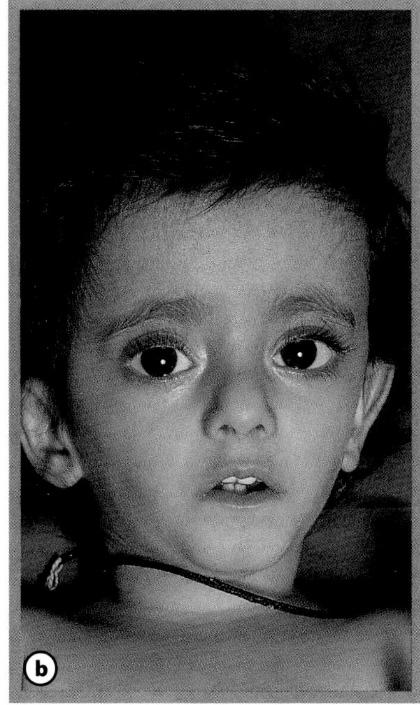

10.5a and 10.5b Russell–Silver dwarfism

This syndrome is characterized by intra-uterine growth retardation, triangular-shaped facies, body asymmetry and clinodactyly of the fifth fingers. There is short stature with a normal growth velocity during childhood and puberty may be early. Trials of growth hormone have so far not shown any advantages in terms of adult height. Some patients have an associated uniparental disomy.

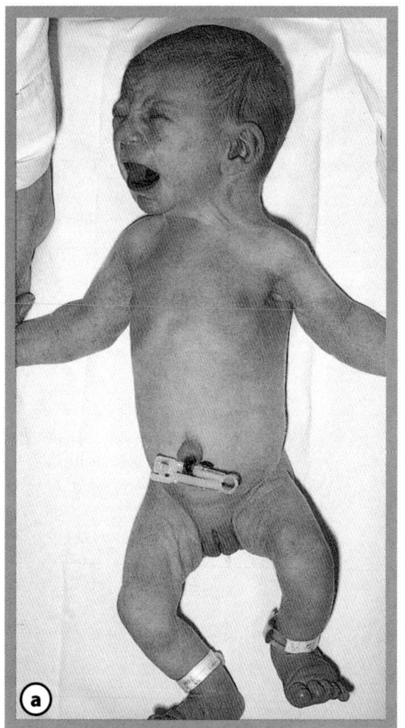

10.6a and 10.6b Turners syndrome (45, XO)
A classical feature of this disorder is a webbed neck with a low posterior hairline. Lymphoedema of the dorsum of hands and feet is a frequently found. The chest may be broad with wide-spaced nipples; cardiac defects, such as coarctation of the aorta, occur in about 20% of patients. Often, an increased carrying angle at the elbow is noted. Up to 50–60% of girls with Turner syndrome have XO karyotype, the rest are mosaic or have deletions of the second X chromosome.

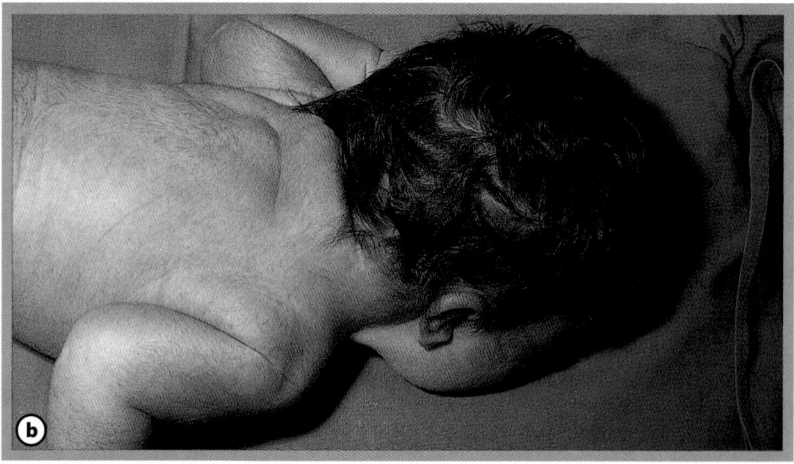

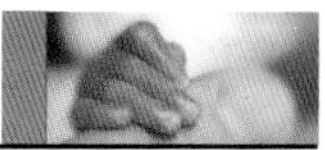

10.7 Potter's syndrome

This condition is caused by renal agenesis leading to oligohydramnios which results in postural deformity, growth retardation and severe pulmonary hypoplasia. The characteristic facial features, also referred to as 'Potter's facies', include large, low-set ears, prominent epicanthic folds and a flattened nose. Resuscitation after birth is usually unsuccessful due to severe pulmonary hypoplasia.

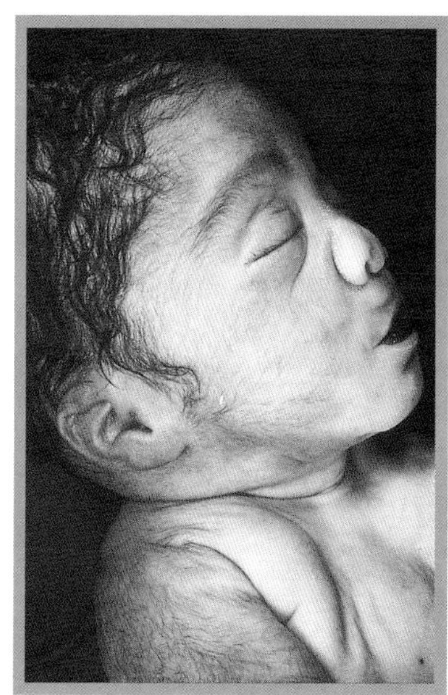

10.8 Robinow syndrome

This is also known as 'fetal face' syndrome. The characteristic features of this autosomal dominant condition are macrocephaly, frontal bossing, hypertelorism, small upturned nose and posteriorly rotated ears. Other skeletal abnormalities are common. These infants often have very small genitalia and cryptorchidism, leading to initial problems in deciding the sex of the newborn infant.

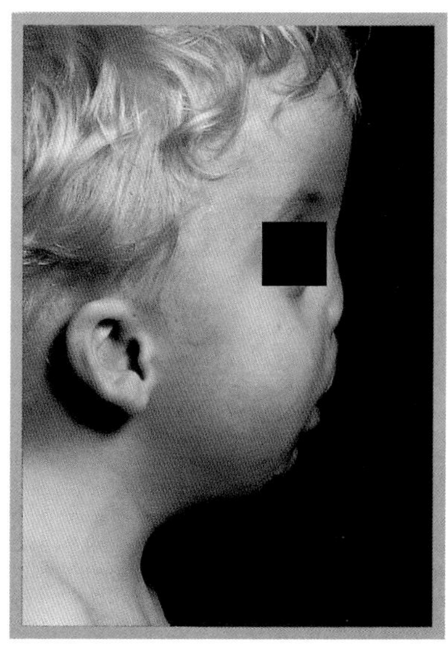

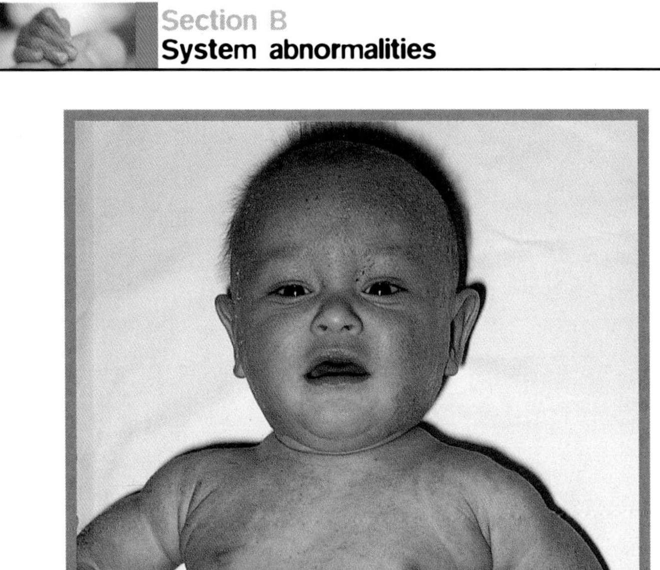

10.9 Wiskott–Aldrich syndrome

This is an X-linked condition with thrombocytopaenia, eczema and immunodeficiency. The underlying cellular defect is as yet unclear. Treatment is supportive. Without successful bone marrow transplant the average life expectancy is around 3 years.

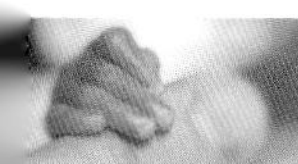

11 Endocrine

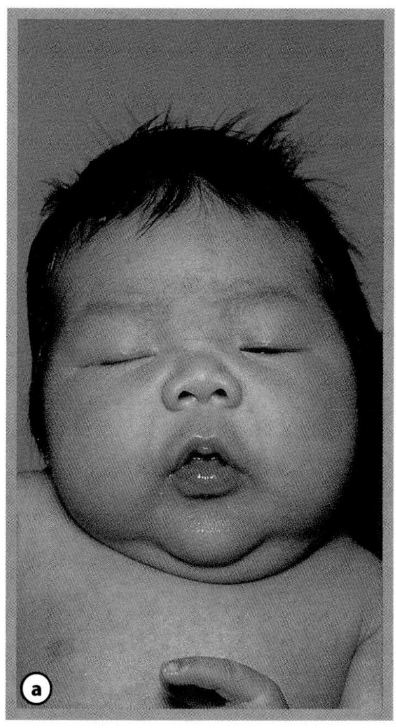

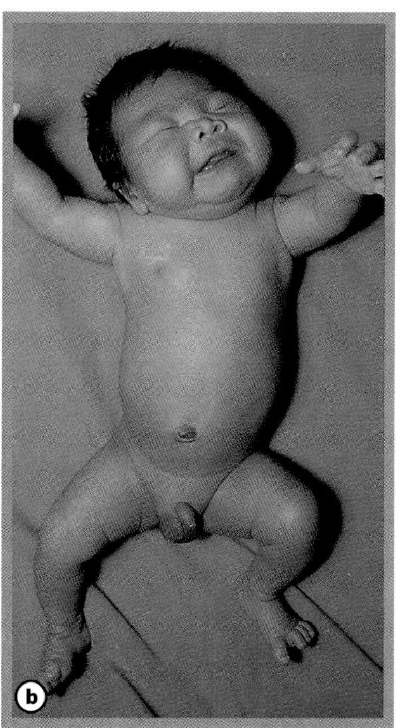

11.1a and 11.1b Congenital hypothyroidism
The severe manifestations of congenital hypothyroidism in infancy have virtually disappeared due to neonatal screening. However some infants may present within the first few weeks of life with prolonged jaundice, hoarse cry and coarse facies as shown in **11.1a** and **11.1b**. Life-long-treatment with thyroxine is required.

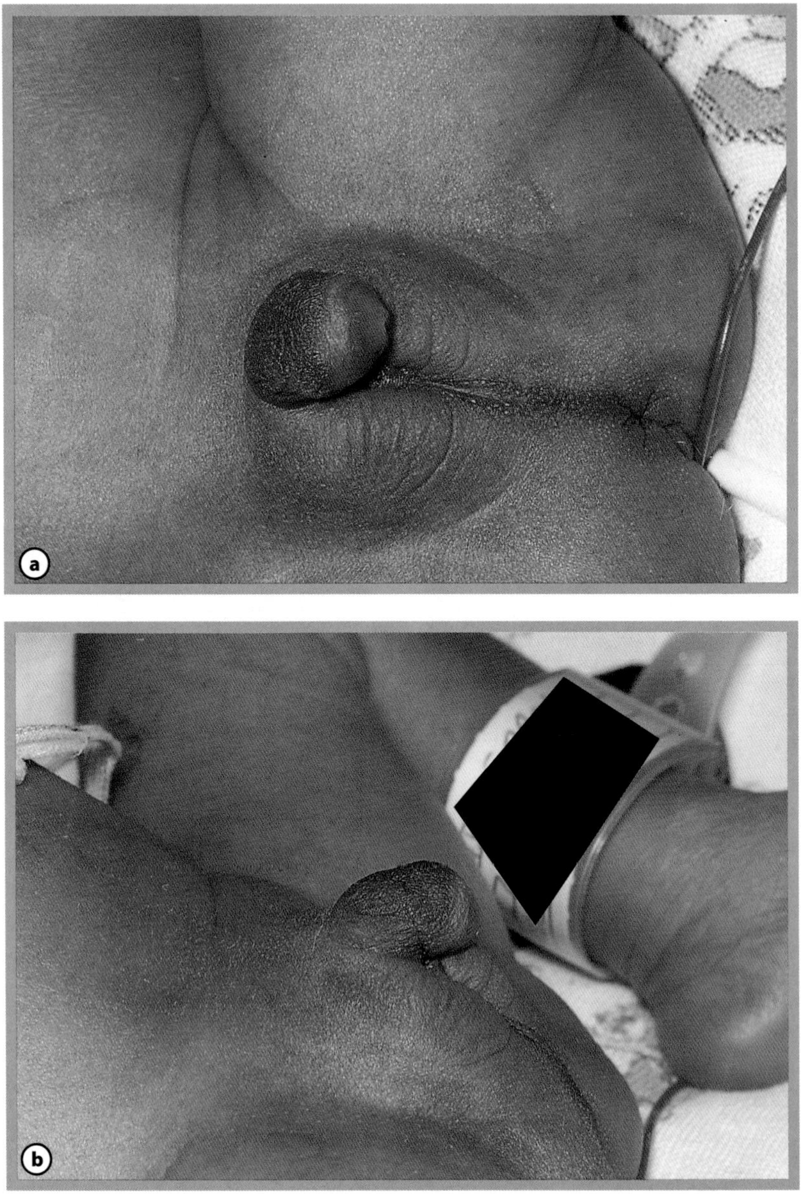

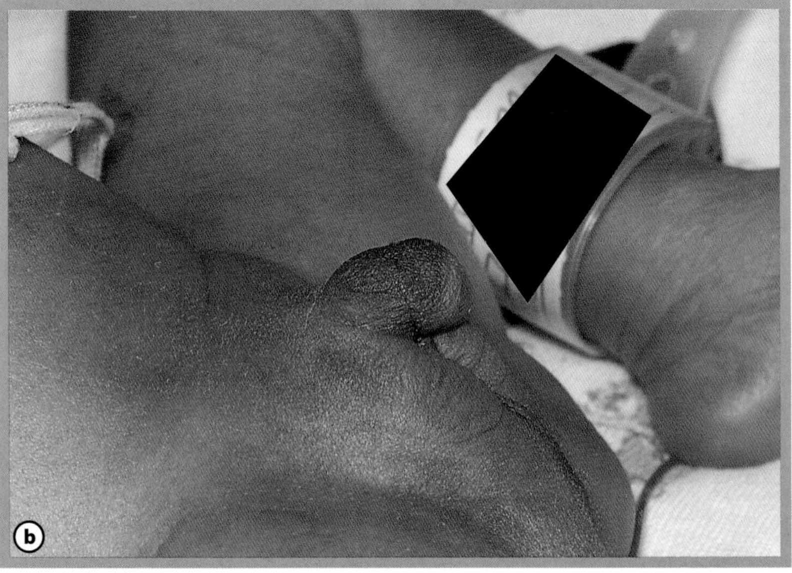
b

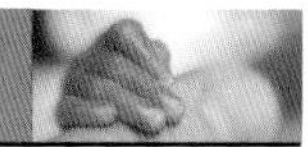

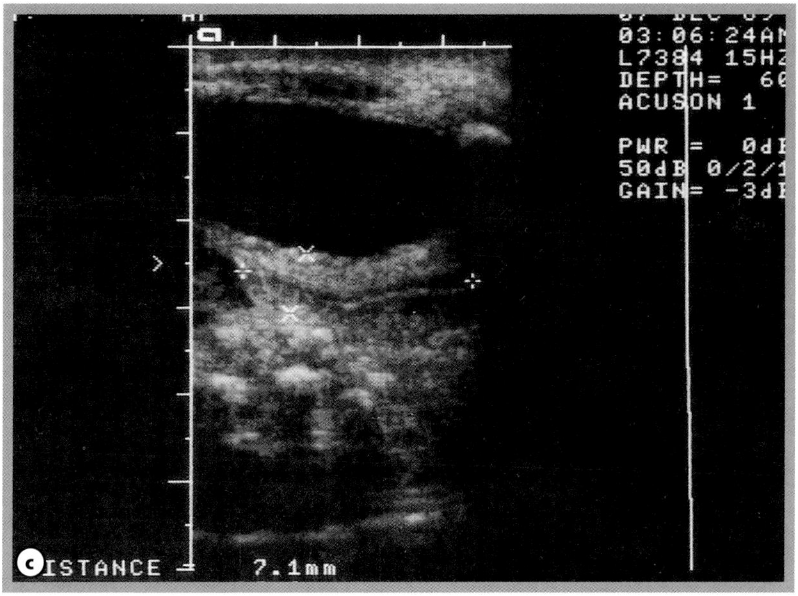

11.2a, 11.2b and 11.2c Ambiguous genitalia

This female infant had marked cliteromegaly and a thickened uterus as shown on ultrasound in **11.2c**. Infants with ambiguous genitalia may be classified as either:

- Virilized female (XX karyotype, normal female internal anatomy and virilization by excess androgens).
- Poorly virilized male (XY karyotype with insufficient androgen action, secondary to pituitary or gonadal defects or abnormalities of the androgen receptor).
- True hermaphrodite (both ovarian and testicular tissue, usually XX karyotype but occasionally XO/XY mosaics).

The sex of rearing depends on the potential for normal function, not the karyotype. The most common cause in the UK is congenital adrenal hyperplasia (virilized female).

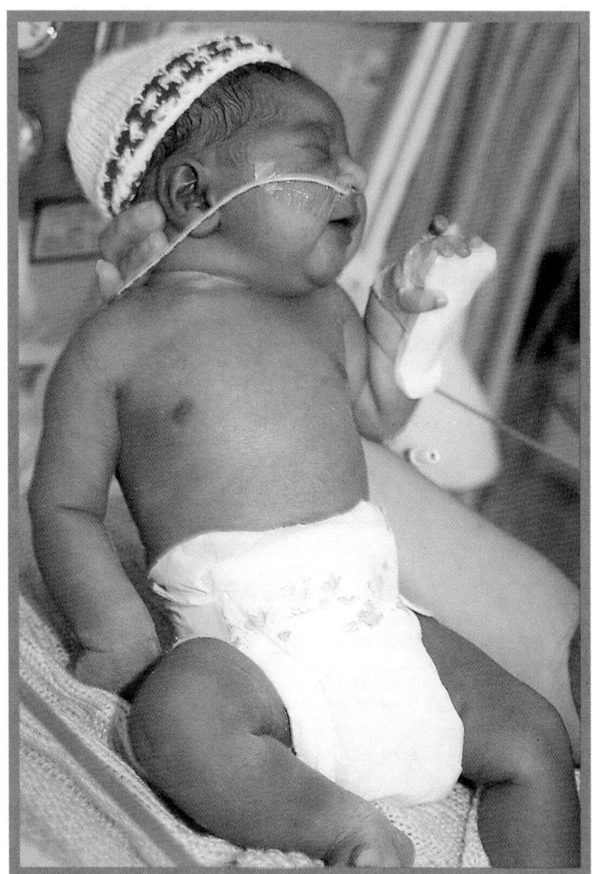

11.3 Infant of diabetic mother
The classical appearance of a large for dates infant caused by *in-utero* hyperinsulinaemia is shown. This is associated with macrosomia and polycythaemia. In addition, there is an increased risk of congenital abnormalities such as sacral agenesis. The main neonatal complication is profound hypoglycaemia. This infant also had an Erb's palsy of the right side.

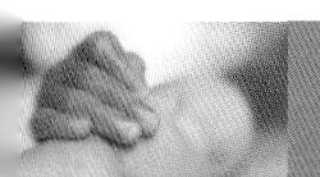

12 Problems particular to the premature infant

12.1 Respiratory distress syndrome

Premature infants are particularly prone to develop respiratory distress caused mainly by surfactant deficiency. This chest radiograph taken at 24 hours of age shows the typical changes of respiratory distress syndrome often described as a ground-glass appearance, characterized by diffuse fine granular opacification of both lung fields with an air bronchogram, highlighting the air-filled bronchi against the atelectatic lungs.

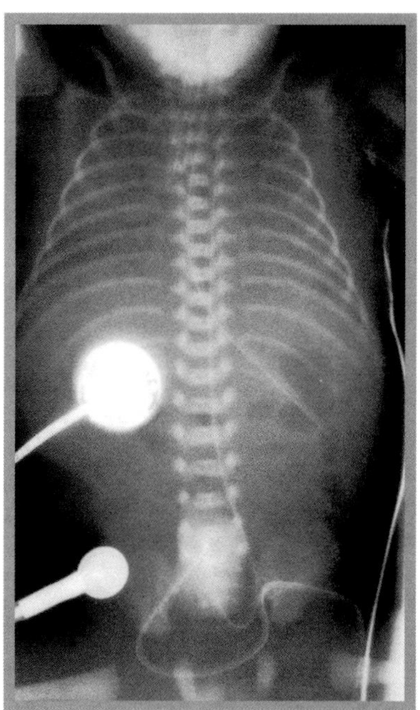

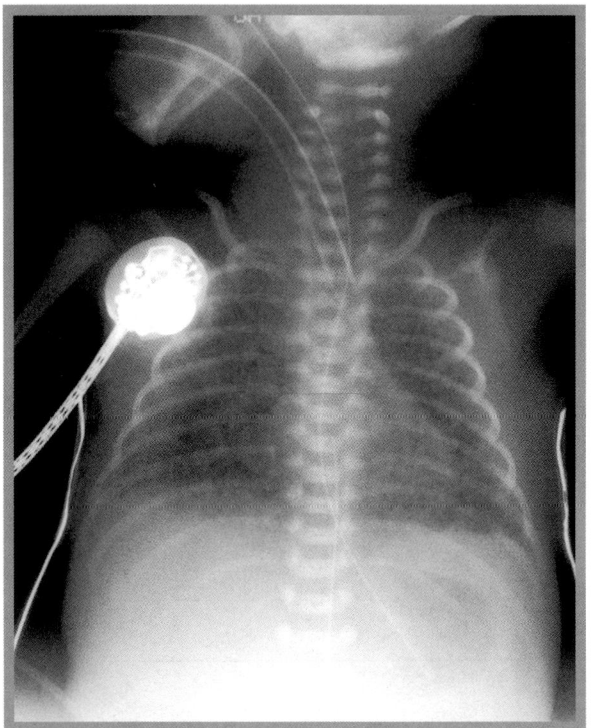

12.2 Pulmonary interstitial emphysema

The appearances on the chest radiograph, diffuse small non-confluent cystic radiolucencies, are caused by air trapped within the perivascular sheaths of the lung. It is predominantly seen in the surfactant-deficient lung after positive pressure ventilation. It is thought that pulmonary interstitial emphysema is a stage before the development of bronchopulmonary dysplasia.

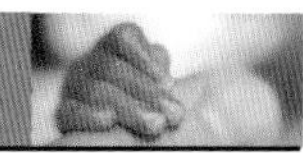

12.3a and 12.3b
Bronchopulmonary dysplasia

Bronchopulmonary dysplasia usually, although not exclusively, occurs after delayed recovery from respiratory distress syndrome (as in this infant). The severity of bronchopulmonary dysplasia is usually judged on both clinical grounds as well as radiographic changes. The old system of grading the chest radiograph changes I–IV is no longer used. The major changes observed on the chest radiograph are hyperinflation with areas of increased density and areas of emphysema. In the pre-terminal stage as illustrated in **12.3b** there is gross overinflation with cardiac compromise.

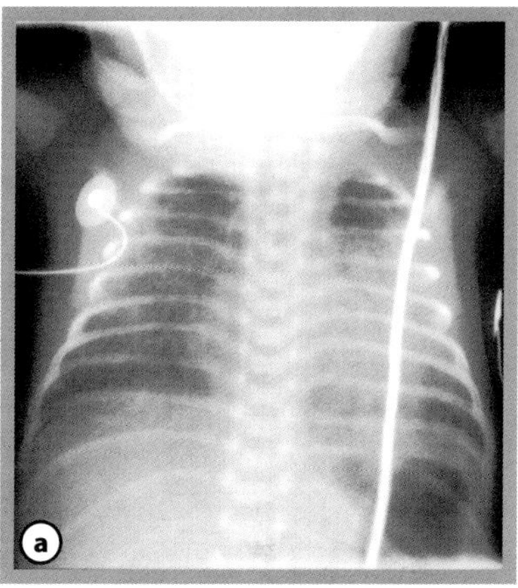

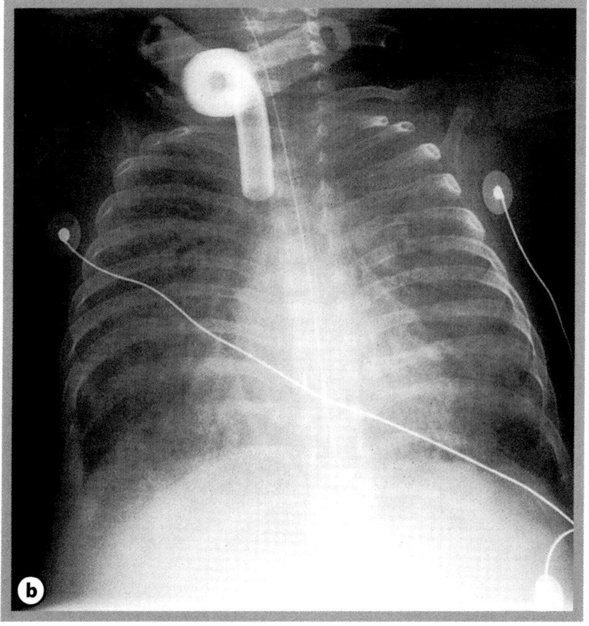

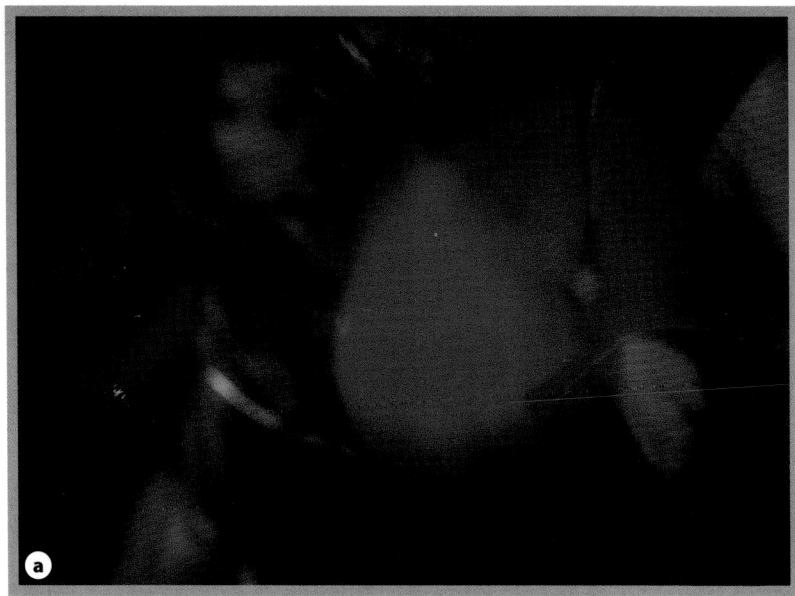

12.4a, 12.4b and 12.4c Pneumothorax

A pneumothorax is more common in premature infants but is not only confined to this group. It is also seen in meconium aspiration as well as occurring spontaneously in some term infants. In this infant it occurred as a result of respiratory distress syndrome. In order to diagnose a pneumothorax a cold light is often used to try to illuminate the affected side as shown in **12.4a**. The chest X-ray in **12.4b** confirms the presence of the pneumothorax. The follow-up slide, **12.4c**, shows the pneumothorax drained using a chest drain. The occurrence of a pneumothorax is associated with a marked cardiovascular response, which may predispose a premature infant to a cerebral bleed.

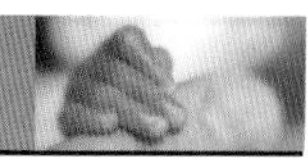

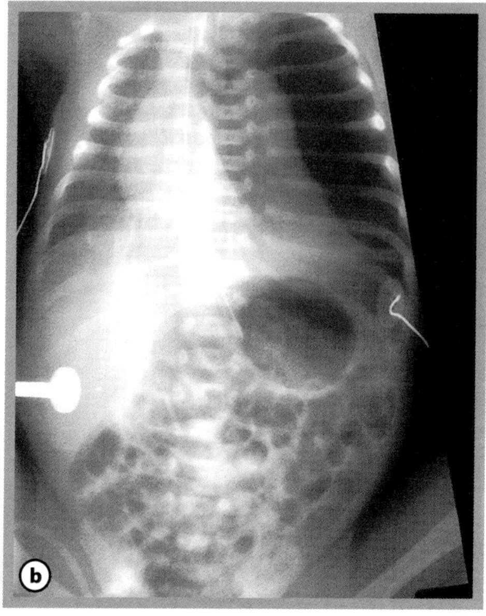
b

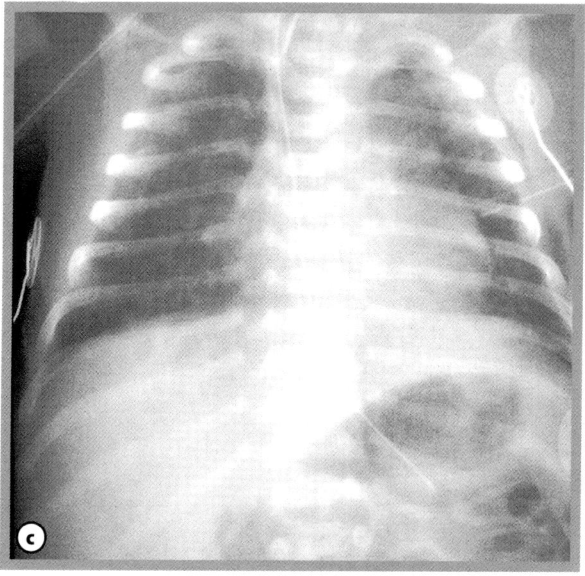
c

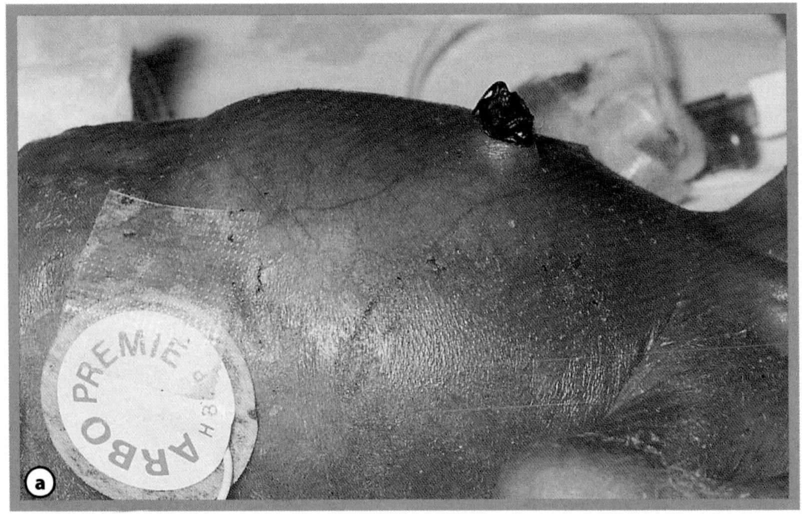

PREMIE
ARBO

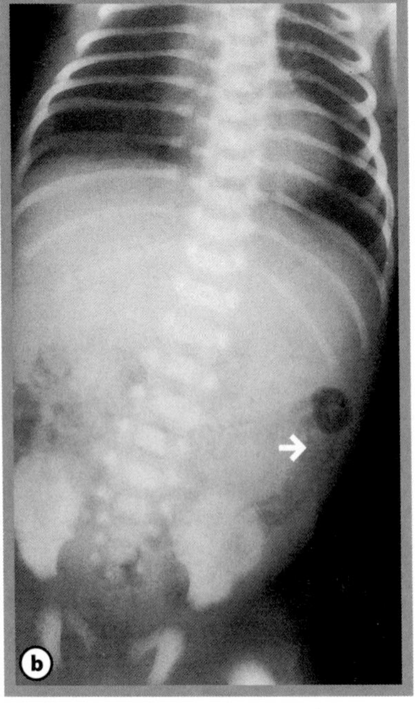

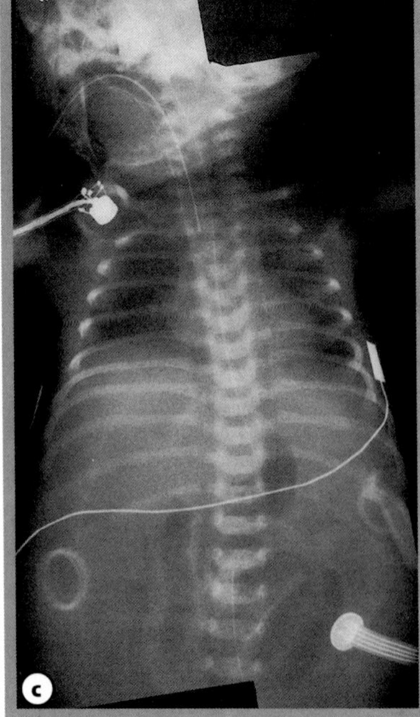

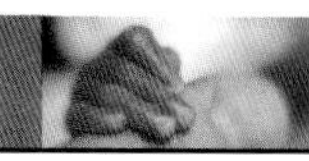

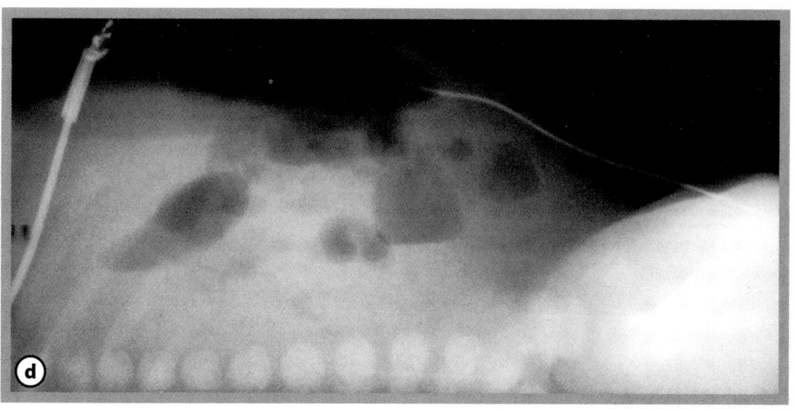

12.5a, 12.5b, 12.5c and 12.5d Necrotizing enterocolitis
This is predominantly a disease of premature infants, particularly those of very low birth-weight. Clinically, the infant often presents with abdominal distension, bilious vomiting and bloody mucousy stools. At a later stage there may blue discoloration of the anterior abdominal wall (**12.5a**). Radiologically, there may be oedema of the bowel wall, intra-mural gas (pneumatosis intestinalis), as shown in **12.5b,** which is pathognomonic for necrotizing enterocolitis. One of the complications of necrotizing enterocolitis is perforation of the bowel. The last two illustrations (**12.5c** and **12.5d**) show clear evidence of centrally placed loops of bowel in the antero-posterior view and free air in the abdomen on the lateral shoot through.

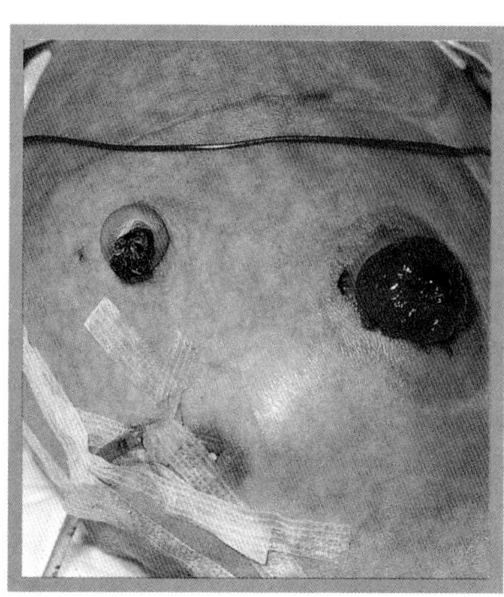

12.6 Ileostomy after necrotizing enterocolitis
As part of the treatment for necrotizing enterocolitis, abdominal resection of the affected part of the bowel may be required. A defunctioning ileostomy is often required when an end to end anastomosis is not feasible.

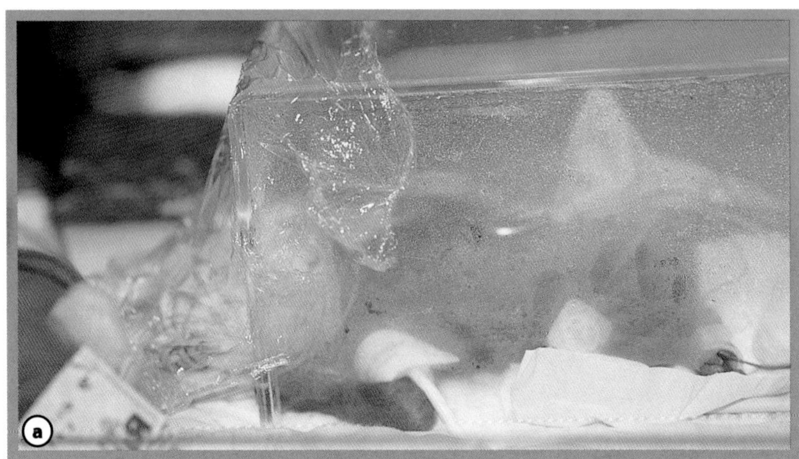

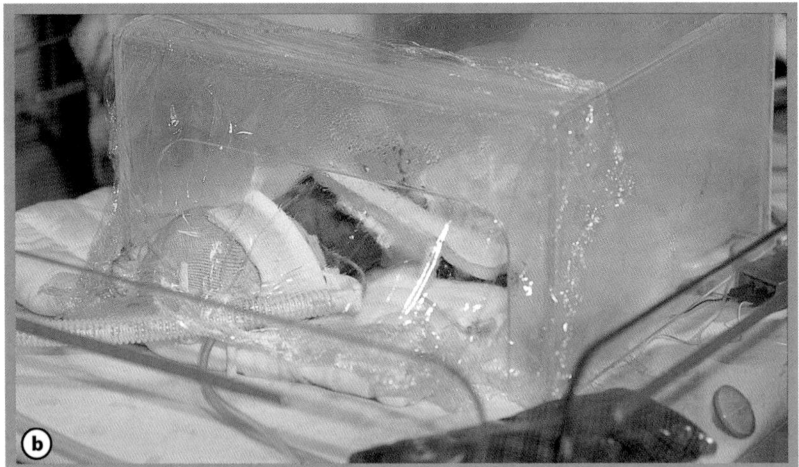

12.7a and 12.7b Skin water loss

Premature infants are prone to dehydration. This applies particularly to very premature infants (26 weeks or less) whose skin is poorly keratinized and thus presents no barrier to transepidermal water loss. A 500 g infant, if not nursed in a high-humidity environment, can lose 10% of his body weight within 90 minutes from water evaporating. This risk can be dramatically reduced by ensuring that the infant is enclosed in a high-humidity (70–80%) environment.

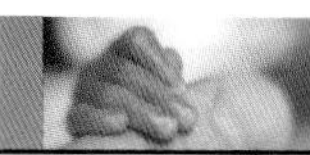

12.8a, 12.8b, 12.8c, 12.8d, 12.8e, 12.8f, 12.8g and 12.8h
Intracranial haemorrhage and ischaemia

Neonatal ultrasound is of paramount importance in assessing the neonatal brain. It is a non-invasive procedure easily carried out at the bedside and provides invaluable assistance for care of the neonate. The major problems facing the neonatal brain are haemorrhage and ischaemia. We feel it to be much more valuable to describe the actual location and extent of the lesion or lesions rather than use some pre-defined label, which invariably may lead to some confusion.

The lesions may vary from a small, unilateral, subependymal haemorrhage to devastating, bilateral, intra-ventricular haemorrhages with subsequent ventricular dilatation and parenchymal infarcts. It is these lesions that may progress to porencephalic cyst formation and subsequent major motor problems. Antenatal or perinatal ischaemia is associated with periventricular echodensities or flares which may progress to the classical multicystic appearances of periventricular leukomalacia. If the ischaemia is extensive and bilateral, there is a very high risk of severe long-term neurological sequelae.

The first two photographs (**12.8a** and **12.8b**) show a saggital and coronal view of a moderately sized, right subependymal haemorrhage, there is minimal ventricular dilatation. This infant made an uneventful recovery. Figures **12.8c** and **12.8d** show the progression from bilateral intra-ventricular bleeds to subsequent ventricular dilatation. Note the time from the first scan to the last scan shown is 22 days. Figure **12.8e** shows an intra-cranial bleed with an associated parenchymal infarct. The follow-up film (**12.8f**) shows the developing porencephalic cyst. This infant suffered from only mild hemiplegia. Finally, **12.8g** and **12.8h** show the aftermath of bilateral parenchymal ischaemia in a 26-week gestation infant, resulting in multiple intra-cranial cysts. This infant has severe spastic quadriplegia.

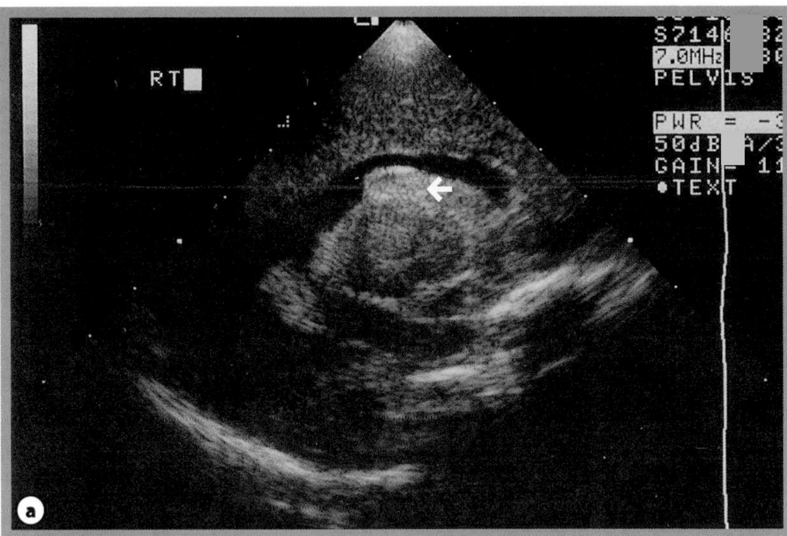

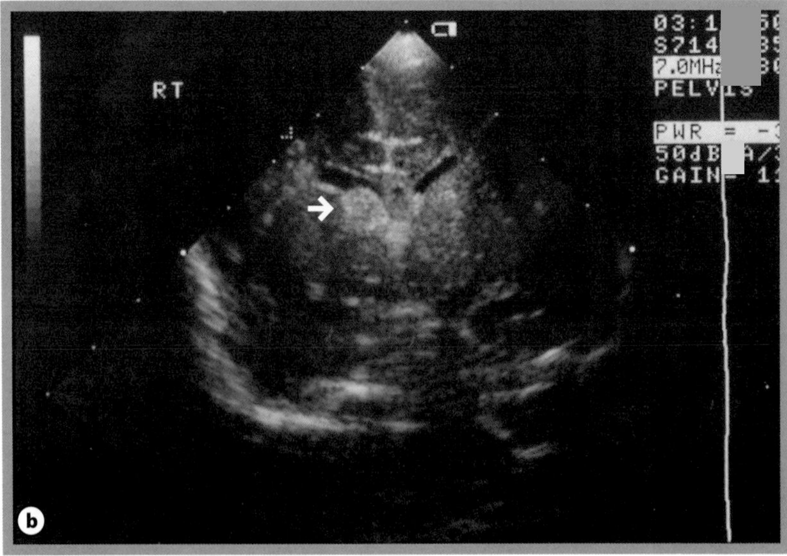

12.8a and 12.8b Subependymal haemorrhage

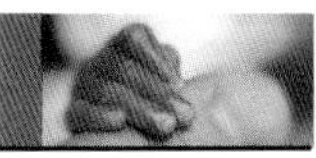

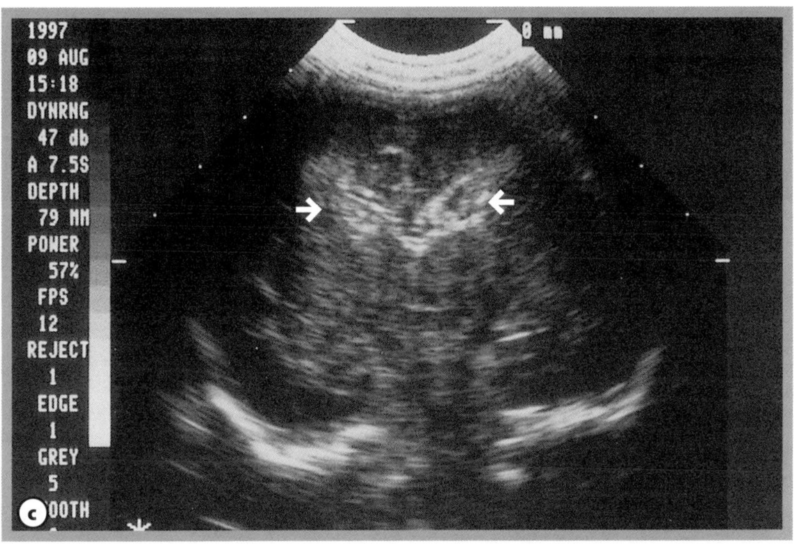

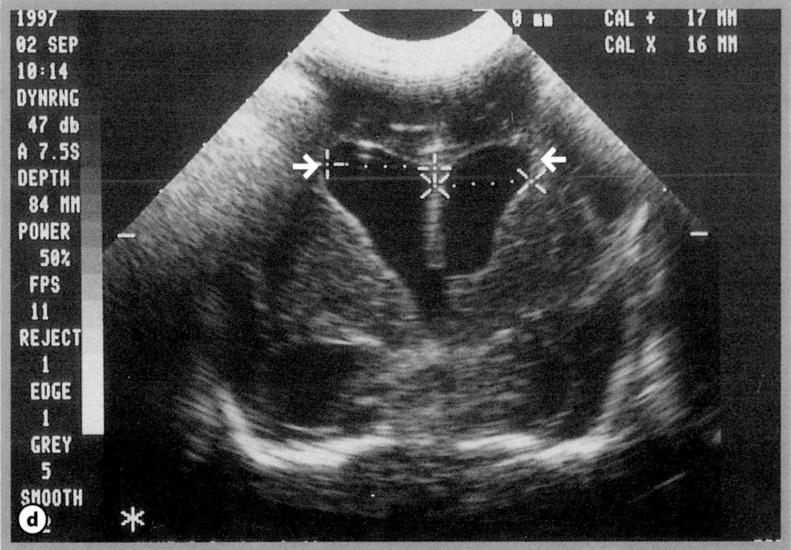

12.8c and 12.8d Intra-ventricular haemorrhage with hydrocephalus

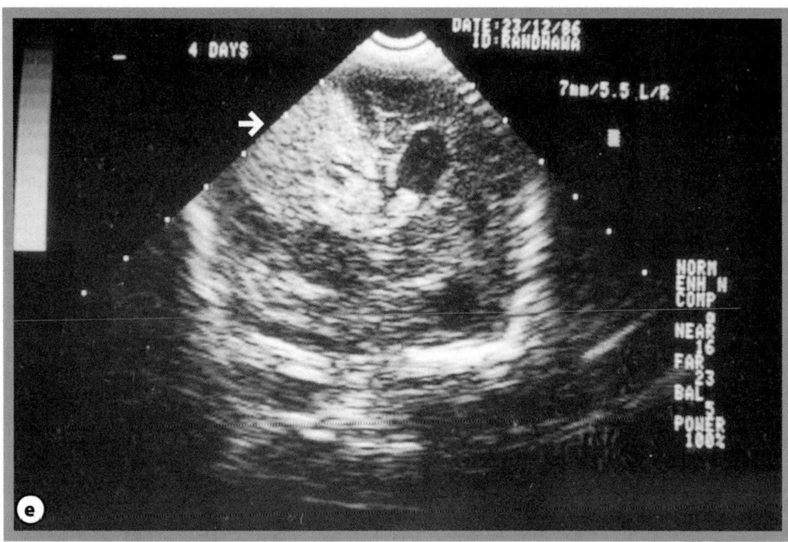

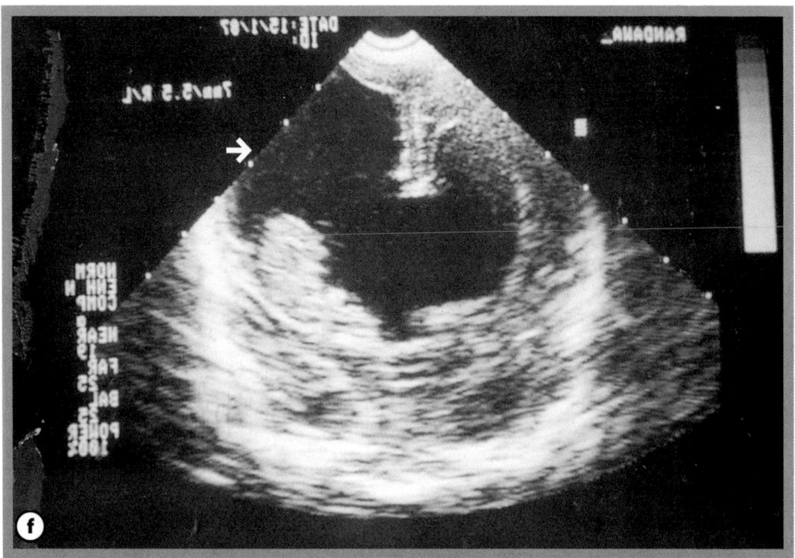

12.8e and 12.8f Parenchymal infarct with porencephalic cyst

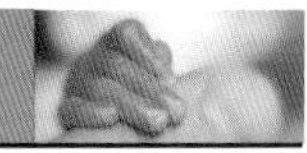

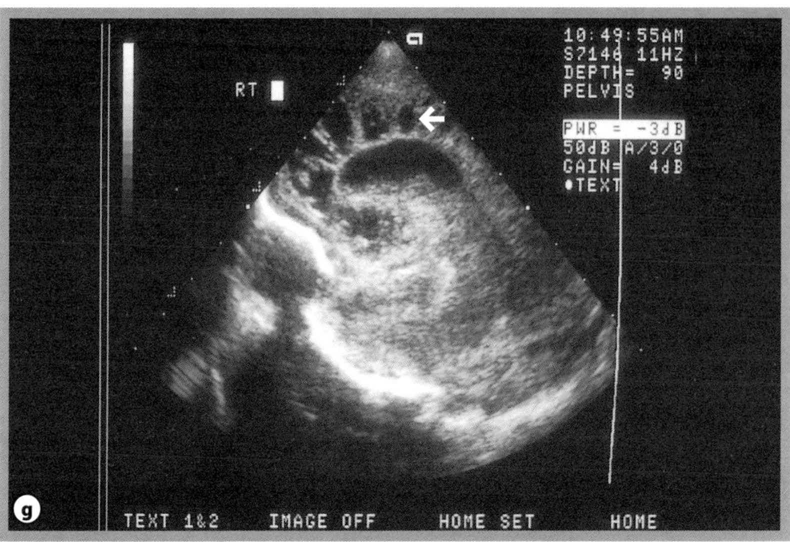

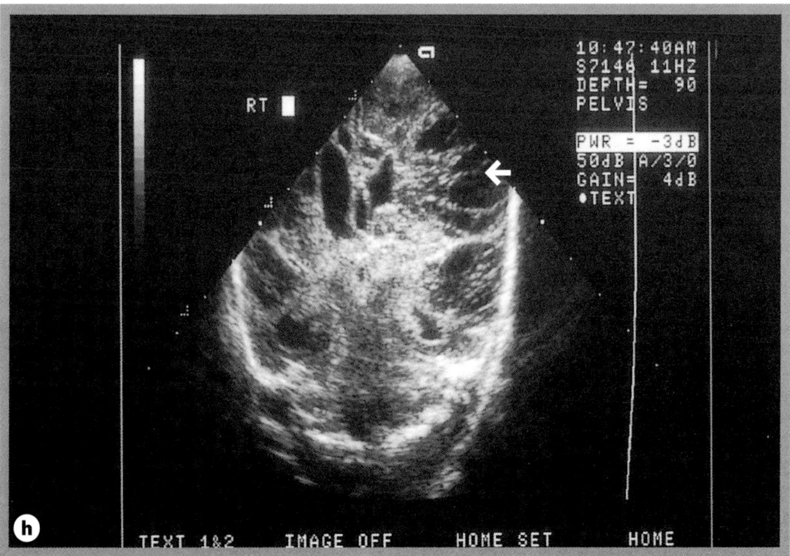

12.8g and 12.8h Periventricular leukomalacia

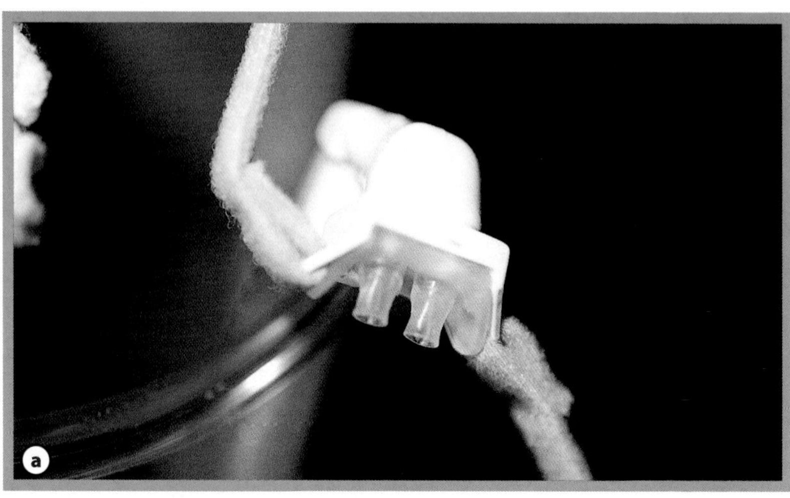

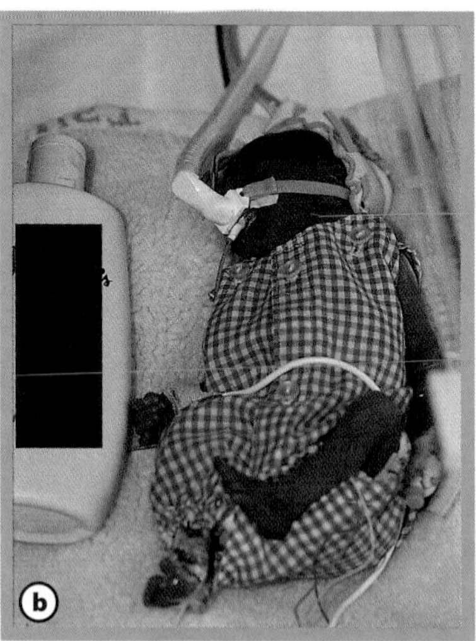

12.9a and 12.9b Nasal continuous positive airways pressure via flow driver
Use of the nasal flow driver has enabled the weaning of very premature infants from full ventilation at a much earlier time than was previously possible. The nasal canula (**12.9a**) fits snugly into the nose of the infant. Care has to be taken when applying the nasal canula as deformity can arise from inappropriate fixing. The infant (**12.9b**) was born at 24-weeks gestation and was immediately oscillated for 8 days before being weaned on to the nasal flow driver.

13 Neonatal tumours

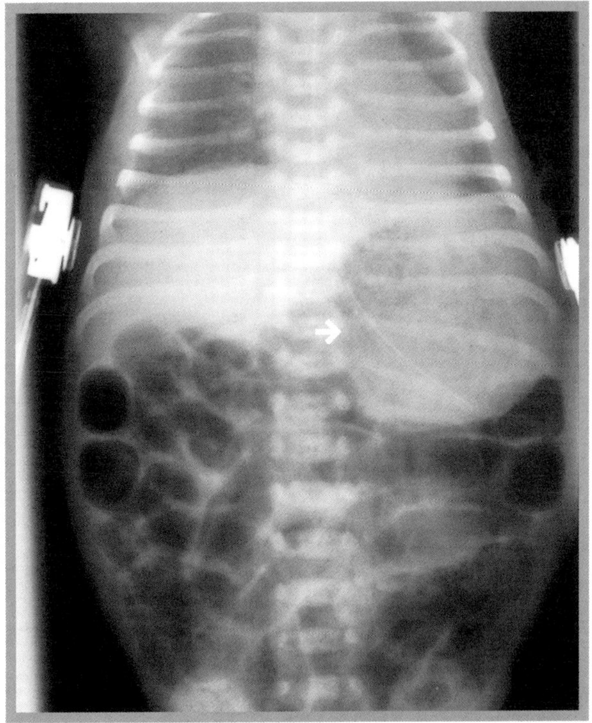

13.1 Congenital adrenal tumour
This infant was noted to have an abdominal mass on routine discharge examination. The radiograph shows the presence of a space-occupying lesion. Further investigation showed the mass to be a neuroblastoma. After a complete resection, this infant made a full recovery.

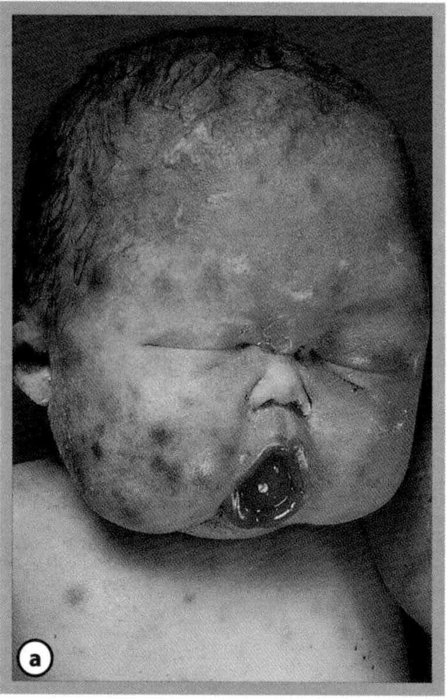

13.2a and 13.2b Neuroblastoma
This tumour may be associated with the development of numerous skin nodules as shown in **13.2a** where, in addition, a large tumour mass is seen arising from the bony structures of the left arm (**13.2b**). The presence of tumours in these sites stages the disease at stage IV. However, if the primary tumour is considered to be at stage I (i.e. there is complete resection without evidence of node involvement) then a further stage, IV-S, is assigned. This scenario usually occurs only in young infants under 6 months and the prognosis is far better than for stage IV.

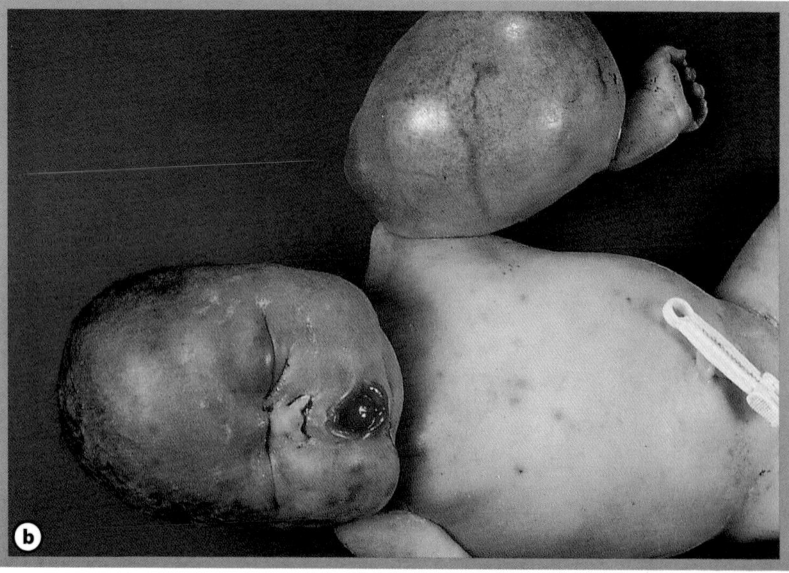

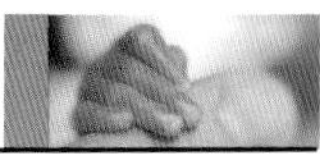

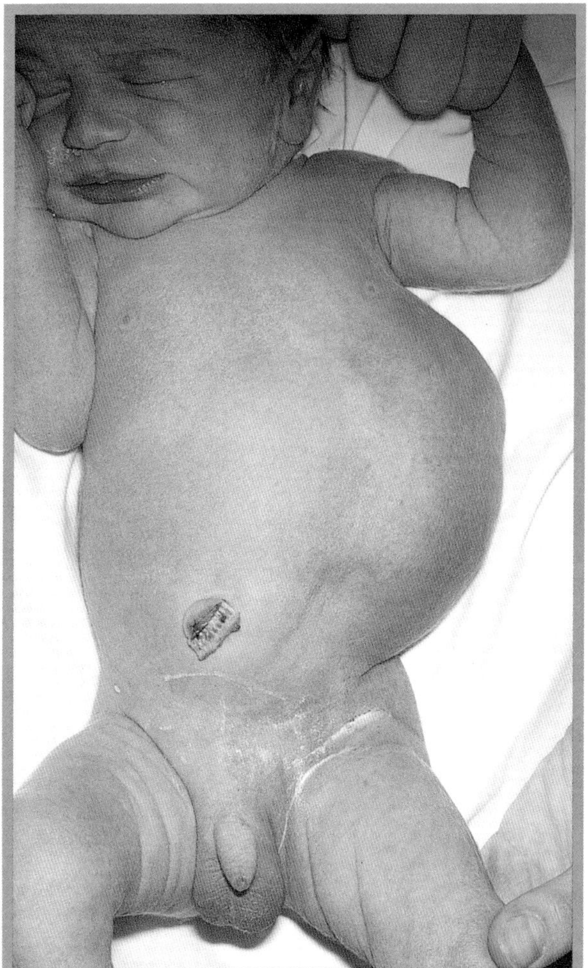

13.3 Congenital renal tumour

This congenital mass was a mesoblastic nephroma which resulted in hypertension, hypercalcaemia and polyuria. It represents a benign tumour in most cases, although there are malignant variants, which may require chemotherapy. Management in this case was complete excision.

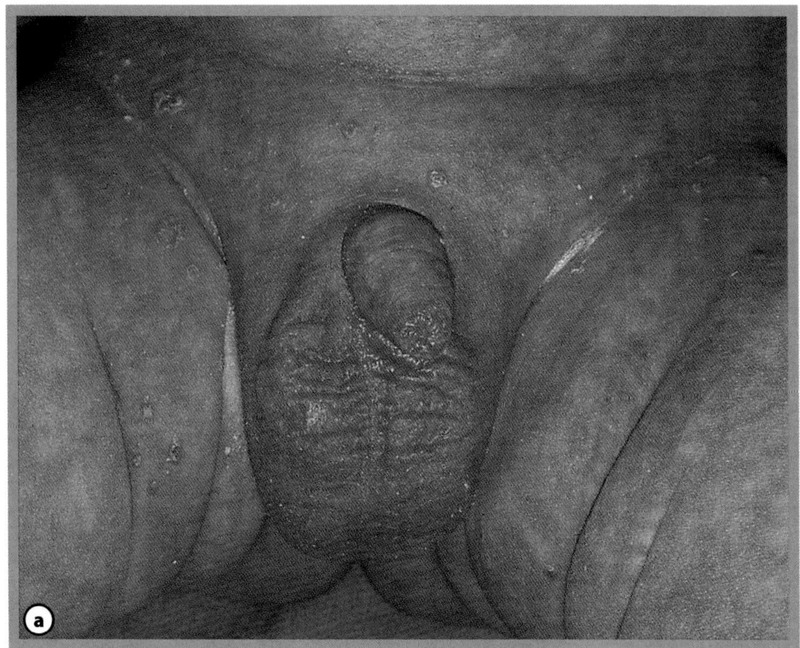

13.4a, 13.4b, 13.4c, 13.4d, 13.4d and 13.4e Langerhans cell histiocytosis
This infant presented at 2 weeks of age with a widespread papular vesico-pustular rash, most evident in the inguinal region. Systemic antibiotics had already been given by the general practitioner and swabs were sterile. A skin biopsy confirmed Langerhans cell histiocytosis and after negative investigations to exclude other system involvement, a diagnosis of isolated skin Langerhans cell histiocytosis was made. As with any single system, the prognosis is good without treatment, although more extensive Langerhans cell histiocytosis disease could develop at a later stage. At follow-up, **13.4d** and **13.4e** show the later development of the classical purpuric lesions in this infant.

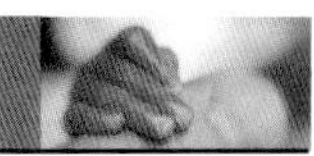

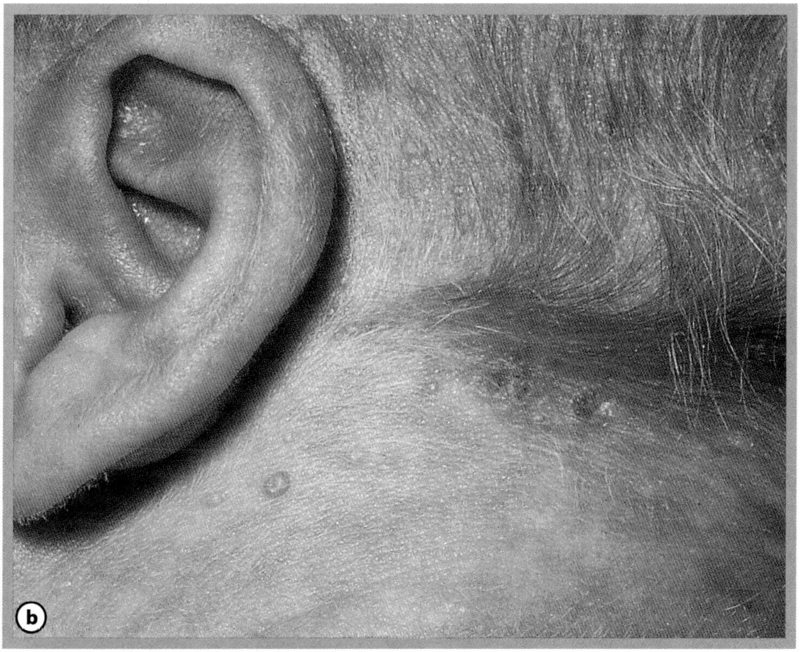

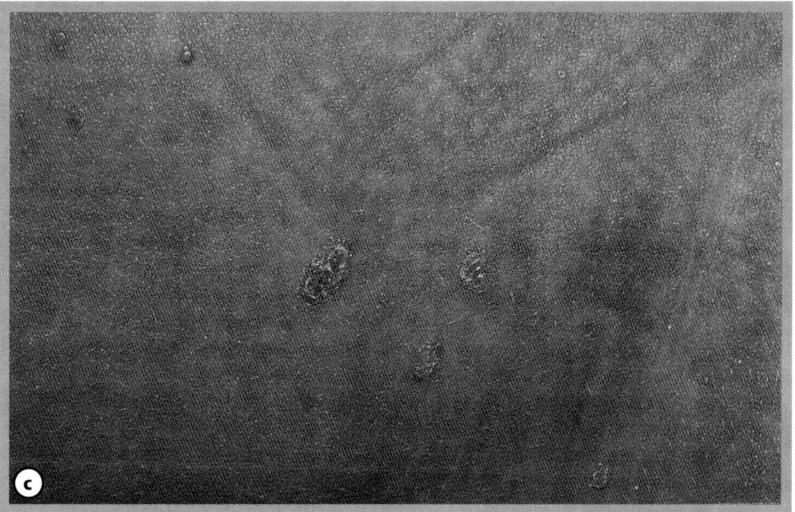

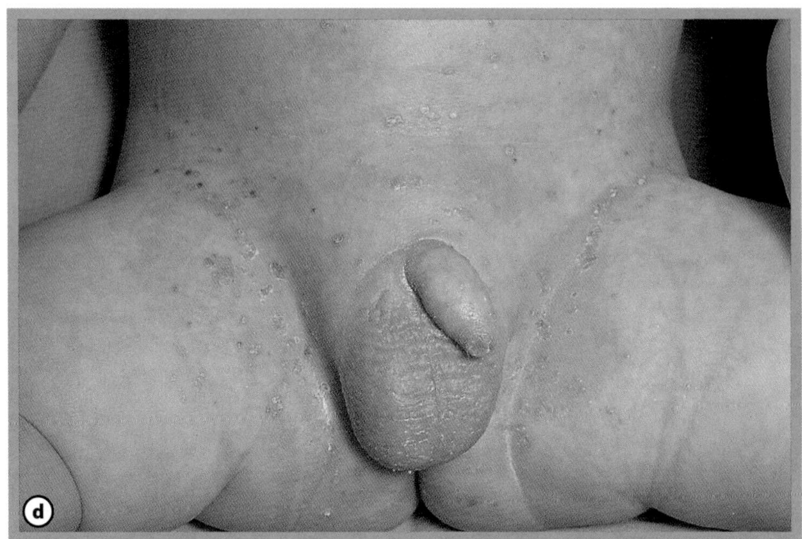

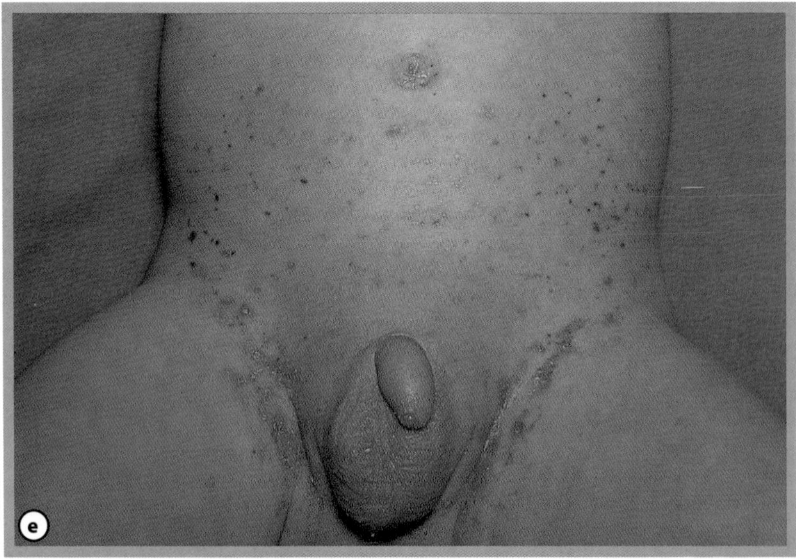

13.4 Langerhans cell histiocytosis continued

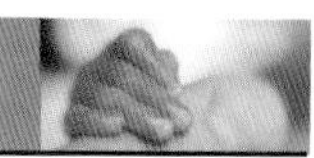

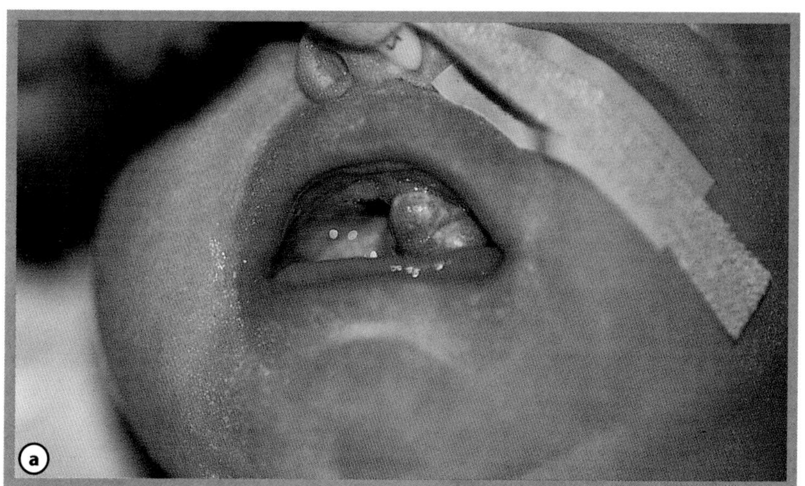

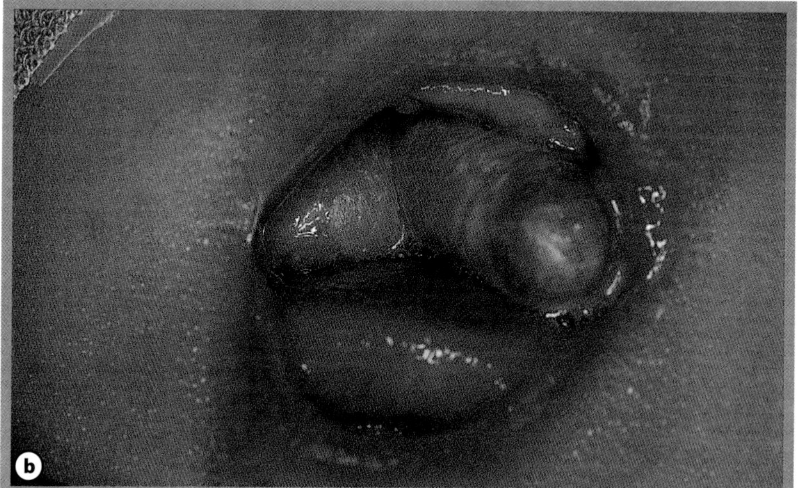

13.5a and 13.5b Pharyngeal teratoma

This infant presented with a greyish lesion protruding from the mouth at birth. There was respiratory distress and the infant was intubated. At laryngoscopy an extensive polypoid mass was seen to arise from the posterior pharynx. Surgical excision was performed and histology confirmed a benign teratoma.

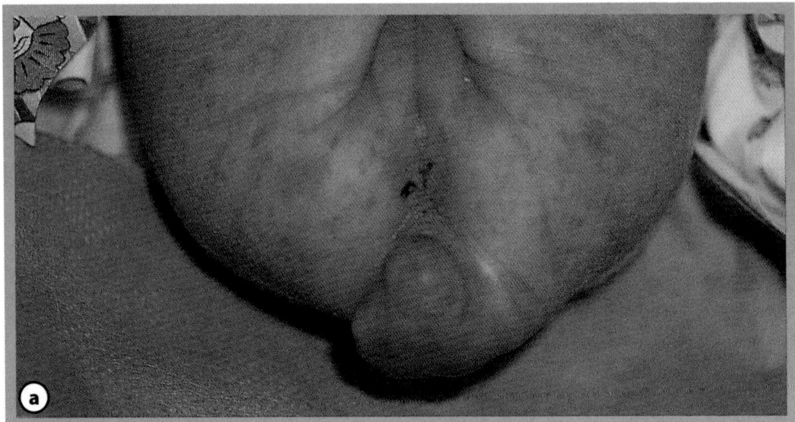

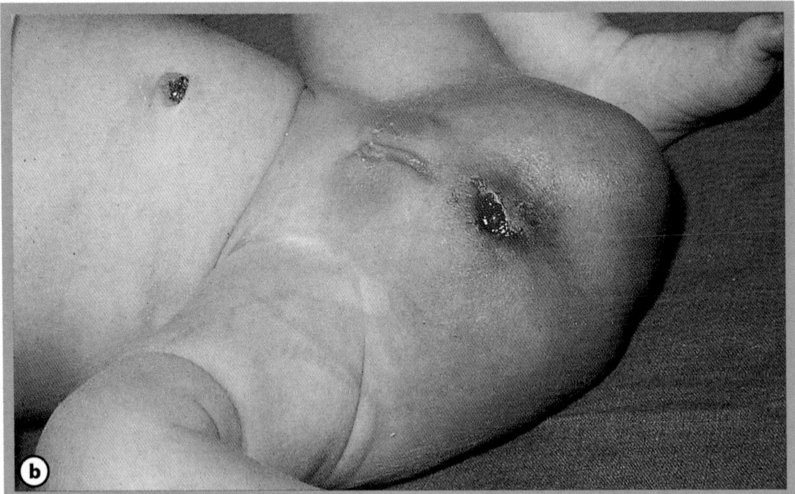

13.6a and 13.6b Sacro-coccygeal teratoma
This is the most common location for teratomas in children, occurring mostly in girls. The classification is based on the site, ranging from stage 1, predominantly pre-sacral, to stage 4, entirely pre-sacral. Treatment is by complete resection and if malignant elements present, adjunctive chemotherapy. The tumour markers, alpha-fetoprotein and human chorionic gonadotrophin, are used as indicators of relapse.

14 Iatrogenic

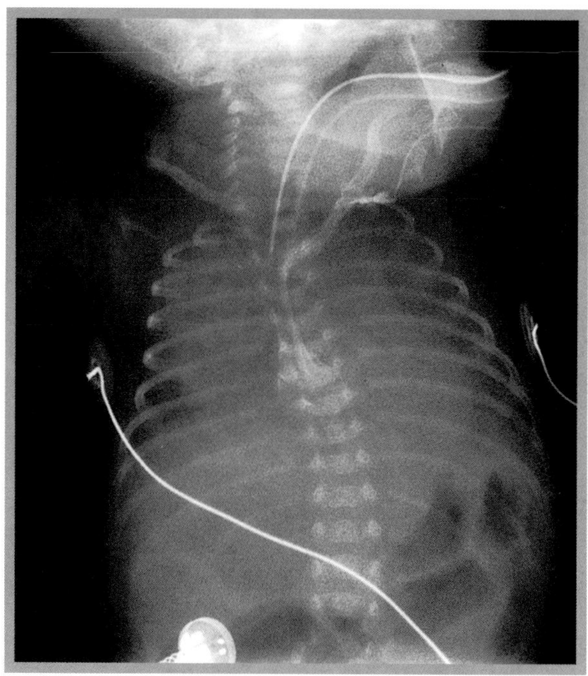

14.1 Excess administration of intravenous contrast material

While checking for the position of the tip of a central sialastic catheter, an excess amount of IV contrast material was administered to this infant. This may result in anaphylaxis with hypotension.

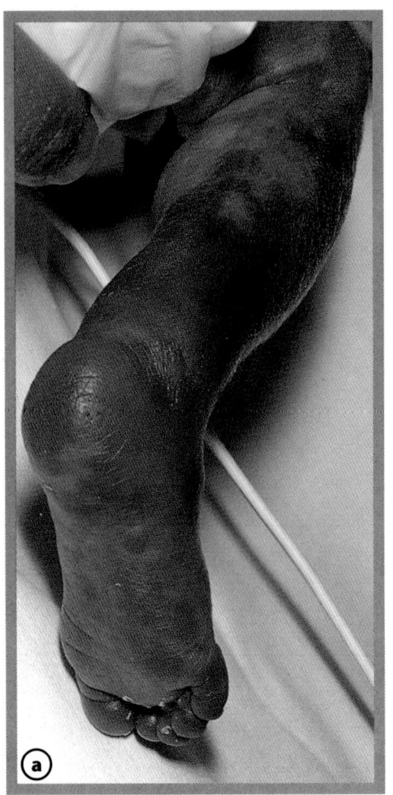

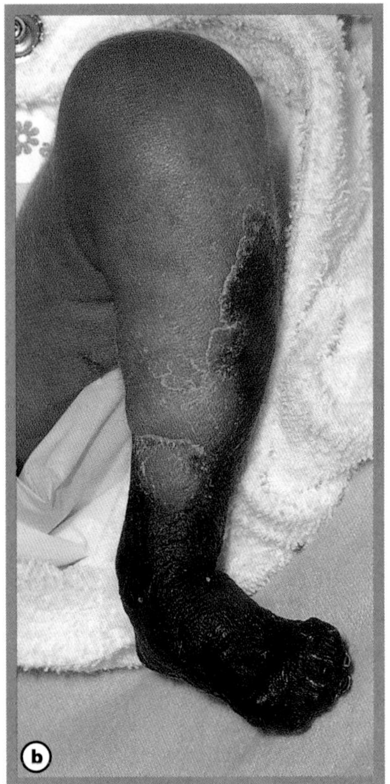

14.2a and 14.2b Gangrene after a posterior tibial artery catheter
The first picture (**14.2a**) shows swelling and cyanosis of the right leg, 4 hours after insertion of a posterior tibial arterial catheter in a 27-week gestation infant which was removed after 10 minutes when the foot became pale and pulseless. The follow-up picture (**14.2b**) taken 2 weeks later shows atrophy and a well-demarcated area of ischaemia. A below-knee amputation was ultimately required. The cause of this rare catastrophic complication was thought to be retrograde embolization of a thrombus.

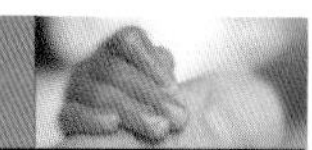

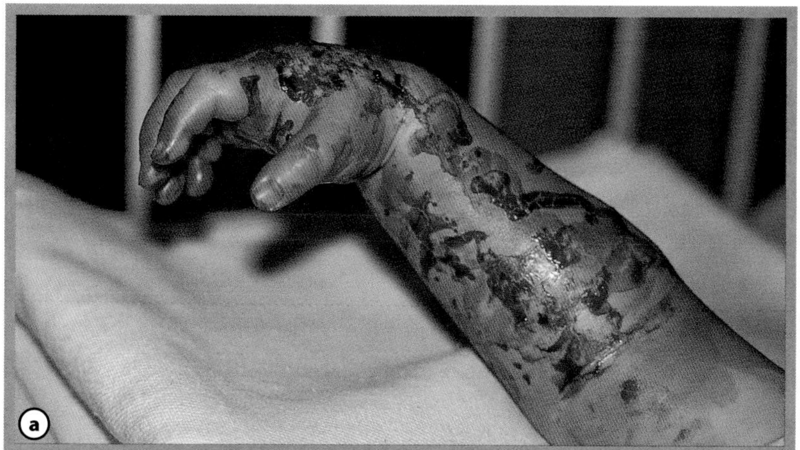

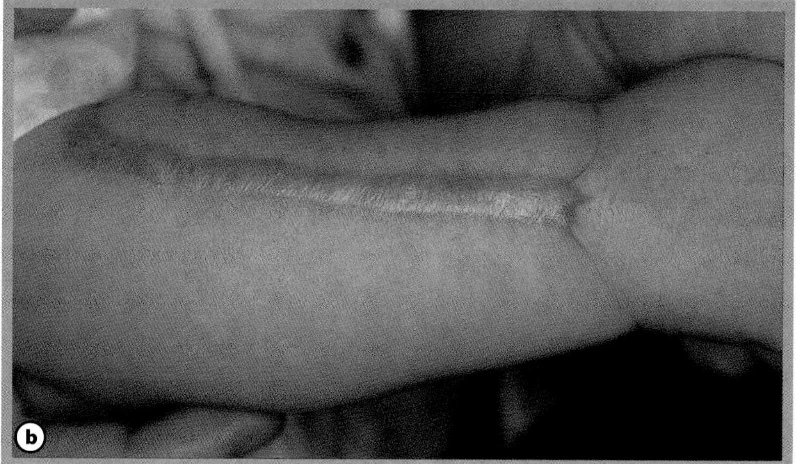

14.3a and 14.3b Compartment syndrome

The first picture shows an acute swelling and a discoloration of a limb after extravasation of dextrose saline fluids from a distally placed peripheral canula. The limb swelled to the extent that the vascular supply was compromised. Acute decompression was attempted with multiple needle punctures but surgical incision was ultimately required. The resultant scar is unsightly but full function of the arm was preserved.

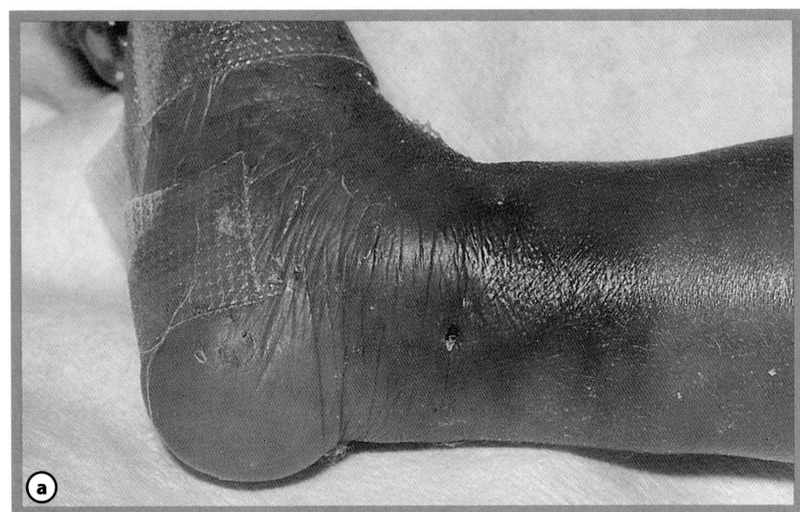

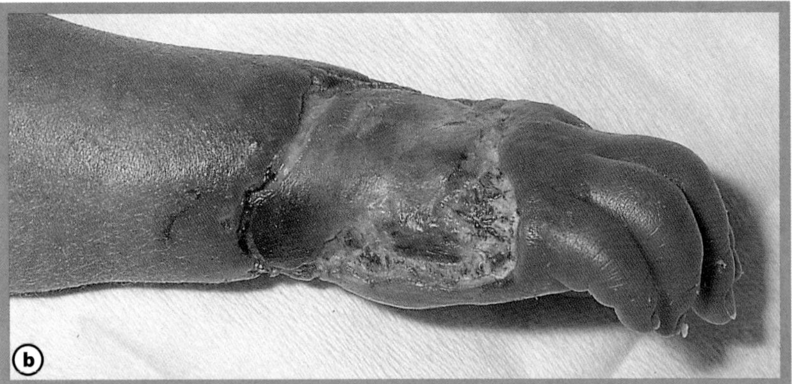

14.4a, 14.4b and 14.4c Total parenteral nutrition burns
This sequence of pictures relating to a total parenteral nutrition burn depicts the early, intermediate and finally the resolving phase, with marked scarring and persisting ulceration. The early stage is marked by swelling and skin discoloration. Once extravasation of total parenteral nutrition is suspected, immediate attempts must be made to minimize the damage by injecting hyaluronidase into the affected areas and then lavaging with saline, allowing escape of fluid through punctured skin holes.

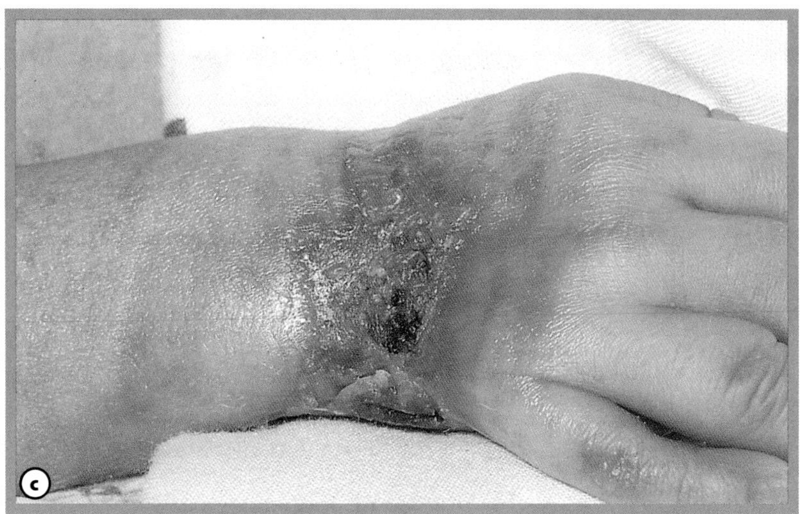

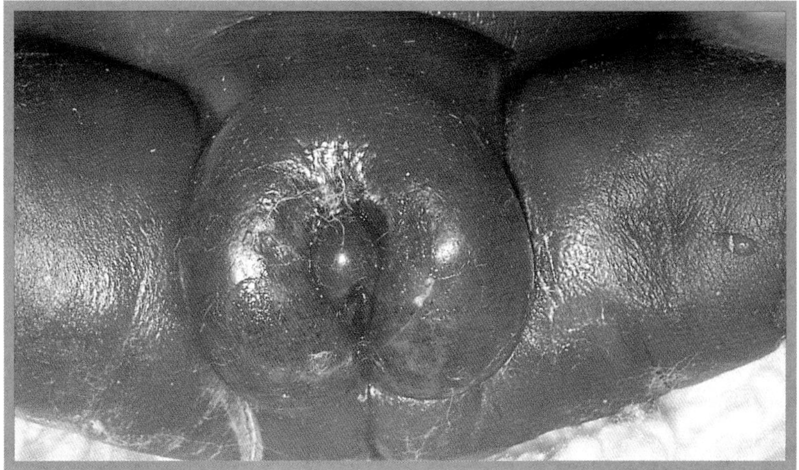

14.5 Vulval oedema

This shows an unusual complication of overenthusiastic fluid administration with diffuse severe swelling of the vulva and underlying tissues. Acute urinary retention occurred.

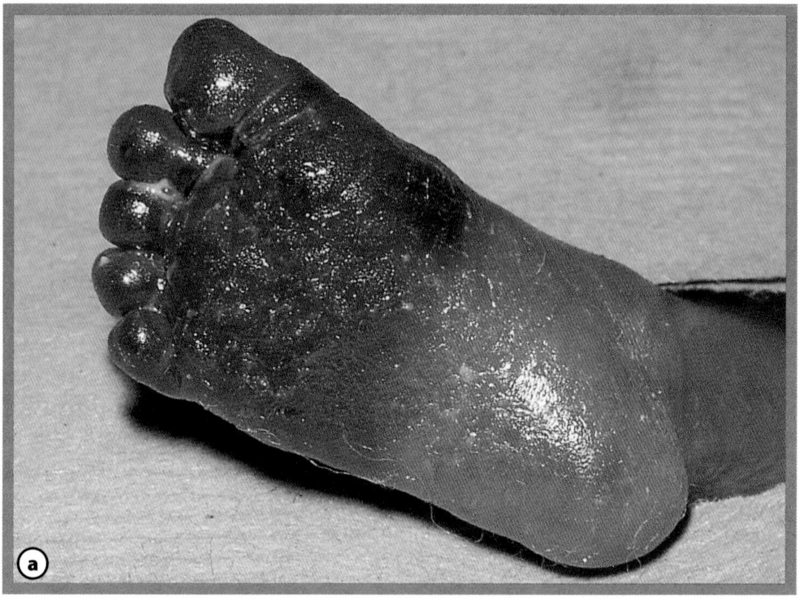

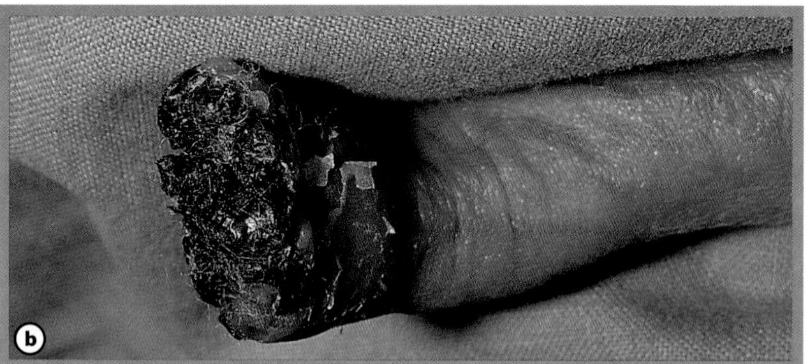

14.6a, 14.6b, 14.6c, 14.6d and 14.6e Ischaemia after an oxygen probe monitor

This injury resulted from an oxygen saturation probe applied too tightly, resulting in ischaemia and ultimate gangrene. A progression through the phases of necrosis, tissue loss and ultimately a good recovery with only partial amputation of toes is shown.

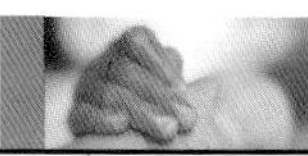

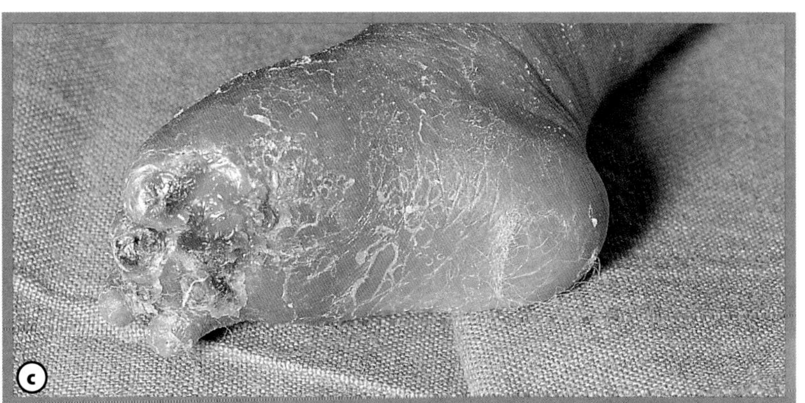
c

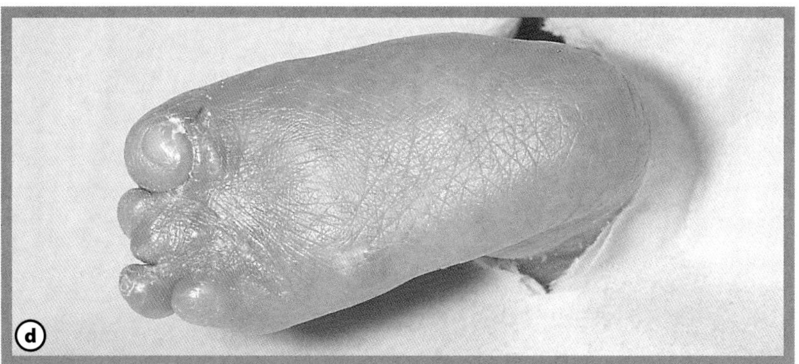
d

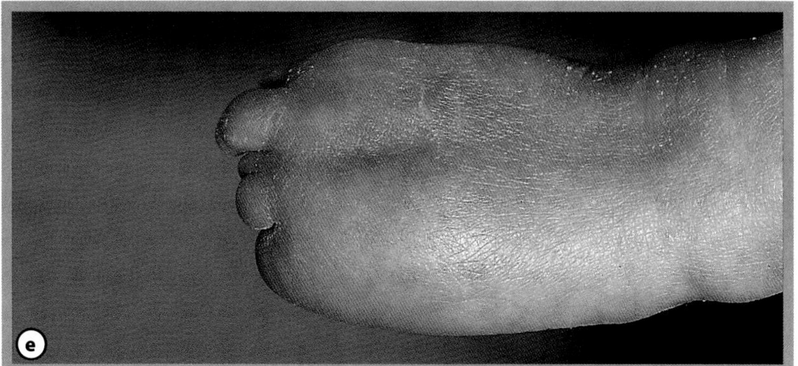
e

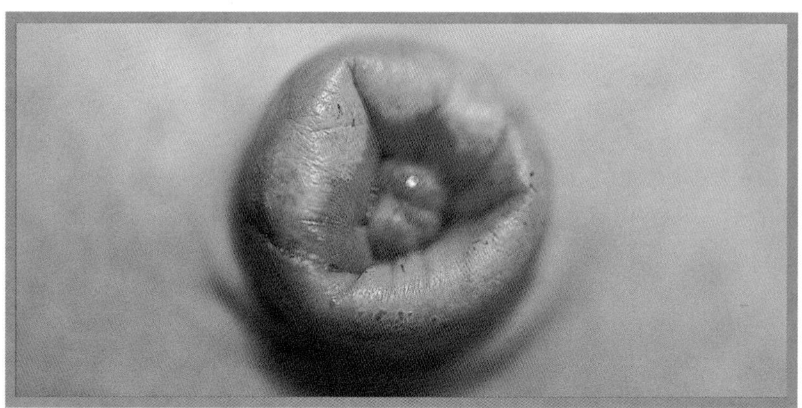

14.7 Silver nitrate burn
In this patient, the umbilical granuloma was treated with silver nitrate. Note the discoloration of the surrounding healthy skin, which occurred as a result of failing to apply a protective layer of petroleum jelly on the normal surrounding skin. Intense ulceration of skin may occur from this error.

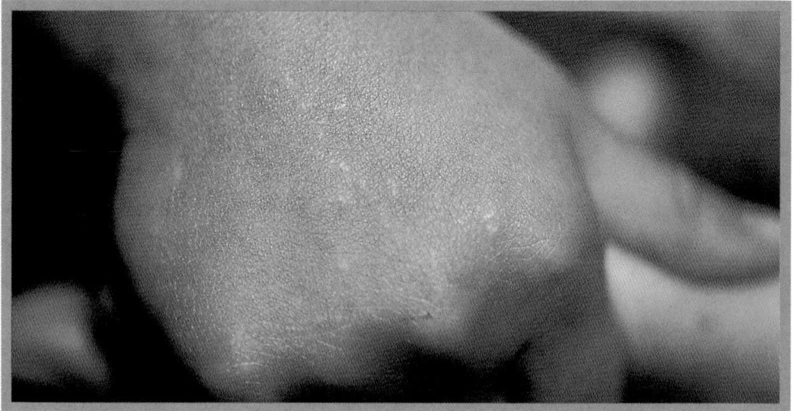

14.8 Hand of an ex-preterm infant
An inspection of the hand can reveal much information. This hand shows the effects of a stay in the neonatal intensive care unit in early life where multiple canulae and venepunctures have left numerous small punctate scars.

INDEX

Numbers are page numbers.

A

Abdominal obstruction, anal stenosis with 108
Acrodermatitis enteropathica 42
Acyclovir
  for eczema herpeticum 40
  for neonatal herpes 46
Adrenal hyperplasia, congenital 149
Adrenal tumour, congenital 165
Albinism, ocular 59
Alpha-1 anti-trypsin deficiency 105
1-alpha calcidol 132
Amniotic bands 118–19
Anaemia, cephalohaematoma causing 1
Anencephaly 76
Angular dermoid cyst 53
Anhidrosis, in Horner syndrome 56
Aniridia
  appearance of 59
  and glaucoma 58
Anophthalmos 55
Antibiotics
  for breast abscess 18
  for eczema herpeticum 40
  for pneumonia 92
  for toxic epidermal necrolysis 37
Antifungal agents, *Candida* infection 12, 13, 16, 17
Anti-Ro antibodies, maternal 37
Anus
  patulous 79
  stenosis, with obstruction 108–9
  web 109
Apert syndrome 125
Arachnoid cyst, congenital 84
Arnold–Chiari malformation 77
Arthrogryposis
  appearance 127
  rocker bottom feet and 122

B

Beckwith–Wiedemann syndrome
  ear crease 142
  facies 142
  macroglossia and 73
Biliary atresia 105
Biliary hypoplasia 105
Birth injuries
  breech hips 7
  caput succedaneum 1
  cephalohaematoma 1
  Erb's palsy 5
  foetal scalp electrode burn 4
  forceps 3
  fractured clavicle 6
  Horner syndrome 56
  ventous extraction 1, 2
Bladder, extrophy, and epispadias 111
Blue spots 30–1
Bowels
  appearance of stools 115
  necrotizing enterocolitis causing perforated 157
  normal pattern of opening 115
Brachycephaly 53
Branchial sinus (cyst) 71
Breast-fed babies
  jaundice 21
  stool appearance 115
Breech presentation
  fractured clavicle 6
  hip displacement 7
Bronchopulmonary dysplasia 152–3
Brushfield spots 54
Buphthalmos 58
Butterfly rash 37
Buttocks, blue spots 30–1

C

Café au lait spots 82
Camptomelic dysplasia 126
Candida (candidiasis)
  oral 17
  perineal 16
  seborrhoeic dermatitis with 12–13
Caput succedaneum 1
Cardiac abnormalities, epidermal naevus 33
Cataract, congenital 57
Cellulitis, staphylococcal skin sepsis 15
Cephalohaematoma 1
Cerebral abnormalities
  and brachycephaly 53
  hypotonia due to 81
Cerebral bleed
  pneumothorax and 154
  see also Intracranial bleeds
Cerebral function monitor 83
Cerebral infarct, twin-to-twin tranfusion causing 19
CHARGE 57
Cherry red spot 54
Chloramphenicol, for conjunctivitis 22
Choledochal cyst 105
Cleft lip 66–7
Cleft palate 68
  and brachycephaly 53
Clinodactyly 143
Cliteromegaly 148
Club foot (talipes equinovarus) 117
Club hand 124
CNS disorders
  epidermal naevus 33
  rocker bottom feet and 122
Collodion baby 32
Coloboma 57
Compartment syndrome 175
Congenital aqueduct stenosis 77–8
Conjunctivitis 22, 61
Corpus collosum, agenesis 85
Cradle cap 16
Craniosynostosis 47
  unicoronal 48–9
Cyanosis 91, 96
Cystic fibrosis, and meconium ileus 107
Cystic hygroma 72
Cytomegalovirus, congenital 43

D

Dacrocystitis 61
Dehydration 158
Dermatitis
  ammoniacal 16
  see also Eczema, Seborrhoeic dermatitis
Dermoid cyst 62
Diabetic mother, infant 150
Disseminated haemangiomatosis 34
Disseminated intravascular coagulation 46
Down syndrome
  appearance 141
  brachycephaly without synostosis 53
  Brushfield spots 54
  duodenal atresia and 98
  and hypotonia 81
  sandal gap 142
  skeletal dysplasia 122
Duodenum
  atresia 98
    in Down syndrome 141
  malrotation 97
  web 97
Dwarfism, Russell–Silver 143

E

Ear
- congenital absence 63
- creases in Beckwith–Wiedemann syndrome 142
- pinna, gross hyperplasia 61

Eczema
- herpeticum 40
- infantile 12, 16, 38–9
- in Wiskott–Aldrich syndrome 146

Edward syndrome (trisomy 18)
- facies 140
- overlapping fingers 140
- rocker bottom feet and 122

Emollients 12, 39
Encephalocoele, occipital 78
Epidermal naevus syndrome 33
Epidermolysis bullosa 36
Epiphyseal dysplasia, multiple 122
Epispadias, bladder extrophy and 111
Erb's palsy 5, 150
Erythema
- annular 35
- multiforme 37
- toxicum 10–11

Erythromycin, for chlamydial conjunctivitis 22
Exchange transfusion 20
Exomphalos 100, 101, 102–3, 142
Eye
- albinism 59
- angular dermoid cyst 53
- aniridia 58, 59
- brushfield spots 54
- buphthalmos 58
- cataract 57
- cherry red spot 54
- choroidoretinitis due to toxoplasmosis 60
- coloboma 57
- conjunctivitis 22
- dacrocystitis 61
- fundus in toxoplasmosis 60
- glaucoma 58
- haemangioma 27
- Horner syndrome 56
- lens dislocation 60
- missing 55
- staphylococcal skin sepsis 14

F

Face
- congenital CMV, 43
- haemangioma 27
- hemifacial microsomia 61
- palsy 4
- port wine stain 28–9
- *see also* Ear, Eye

Facies
- collodion baby 32
- congenital hypothyroidism 147
- cyanosis 91
- Down syndrome 141
- Edward syndrome 140
- fetal alcohol syndrome 139
- neonatal lupus 37
- Pierre Robin sequence 69
- Robinow syndrome 145
- Treacher Collins syndrome 65

Fallot's tetralogy 91
Female, virilized 149
Fetal alcohol syndrome 139
Fetal face (Robinow) syndrome 145
Fetofetal transfusion, acute 20
Fits, congenital arachnoid cyst 84
Flow driver, nasal CPAP via 164
Flucloxacillin, staphylococcal skin sepsis 14
Foetal scalp electrode burn 4
Foot
- cellulitis 15
- rocker bottom 122

Forceps delivery
- facial palsy 4
- marks 3

Fractures
- clavicle, birth-related 6
- congenital humerus 131
- in osteogenesis imperfecta, 130–1
- ricket-related 132
- skull, and cephalohaematoma 1

G

Galactosaemia 21
Gastrointestinal disorders
- duodenal atresia 98
- duodenal web 97
- exomphalos 102–4
- gastroschisis 100
- meconium ileus 106–7
- umbilical granuloma 101
- umbilical hernia 100–1
- vitello-intestinal duct, persistent 99

Gastroschisis 100
Genitalia, ambiguous 148–9
Genitourinary disorders
- bilateral hydrocoeles 116
- bladder extrophy and epispadias 111
- hypospadias 112–13
- inguinal hernia 111

Glaucoma, congenital 58
Glossoptosis 69
Glucose-6-phosphate dehydrogenase deficiency 21
Goldenhar syndrome 64
Great arteries, transposition, cyanosis due to 91
Gynaecomastia 18, 22

H

Haberman test 70
Haemangiomas
- capillary 28–9
- cavernous 24–5
- extensive 26–7

Hand
- ex-preterm infant 180
- paronychia 15

Head
- cleft lip 67
- cleft palate 68
- hemifacial microsomia 61
- misshapen, ventouse extraction 2
- scaphocephaly 47
- unicoronal craniosynostosis 48–9
- *see also* Face, Neck, Neurology, Skull

Head and neck
- cystic hygroma 72
- sternomastoid tumour 72

Hemifacial microsomia 61
Hepatitis 105
- infant of mother with 35

Hepatosplenomegaly
- and congenital CMV, 43
- and congenital varicella 45
- lupus syndrome causing 37
- in neonatal herpes 46

Hermaphrodite, true 149
Hernia
- bilateral inguinal 111
- diaphragmatic 88–9
- umbilical 100–1

Herpes, neonatal 46
High-frequency oscillation 94
Hips
- breech 7
- congenital dislocation 7
  - and metatarsus adductus varus 121

Homocystinuria 60
Horner syndrome 56
Humerus, congenital fracture 130
Hydrocephalus, post-haemorrhagic 77
Hydrocoeles, bilateral 116
Hydrops foetalis 90
Hyperinsulinaemia, in utero 150

Hypoglycaemia
infant of diabetes mother 150
neonatal 142
Hypophosphataemia, neonatal rickets due to 132
Hypothyroidism
congenital 147
and hypotonia 81
jaundice due to 21
Hypotonia 81
agenesis of corpus collosum causing 85
Hypoxia, ischaemic damage to basal ganglia 84

I

Iatrogenic disorders
compartment syndrome 175
excess intravenous contrast material 173
hand of ex-preterm infant 180
ischaemia after oxygen probe monitor 178–9
silver nitrate bur 180
tibial artery catheter, gangrene 174
total parenteral nutrition burns 176
vulval oedema 177
Ileostomy, after necrotizing enterocolitis 157
Inborn errors of metabolism
and hypotonia 81
jaundice 105
Incontinentia pigmenti 33
Inguinal hernia, bilateral 111
Intracranial bleeds 159–63
Intracranial pathology, and incontinentia pigmenti 33
Intracranial vascular anomalies, and port wine stains 29
Intraocular tumours 58
Intravenous contrast material, excess administration 173
Intraventricular bleeds, multiple cysts secondary to 85

J

Jaundice 105
caput succedaneum causing 1
cephalohaematoma causing 1
congenital hypothyroidism 147
discussion 21
twin-to-twin tranfusion causing 19
Joint movement, intrauterine restriction 127

K

Kasabach–Merritt syndrome 27
Klippel–Trenaunay syndrome 29

L

Langerhans cell histiocytosis 168–70
Laser therapy, for port wine stains 28–9
Legs
bowed, rickets causing 132
congenital melanocytic naevus 24
Limb hypertrophy, and port wine stains 29

M

Macroglossia 73
Macrosomia, infant of diabetes mother 150
Male, poorly virilized 149
Mandible
poor development in Pierre Robin 69
underdevelopment 61
Marfan syndrome 60
Mastitis 22
Meconium
aspiration 95
pneumothorax after 154
ileus 107
passage 115
in utero 115
Meningioma 82
Meningitis, neonatal 77
Meningocoele, cranial 78
Metatarsus adductus varus 121
Microcephaly 75
schizencephaly leading to 86
Milia 9
Milk allergy 41
Miosis, in Horner syndrome 56
Mucous membrane disorders
acrodermatitis enteropathica 42
Candida infections 13, 16–17
mucous retention cyst 17
Mucous retention cyst 17
Myelodysplasia 122
Myelomeningocoele
thoracic 80
thoracolumbar 79

N

Naevi
bathing trunk 23
congenital melanocytic 24
congenital pigmented 30
epidermal 33
strawberry 24–5
Napkin dermatitis 12
Nasal continuous positive airways pressure, via flow driver 164
Neck
branchial sinus 71
tracheostomy 70
Necrotizing enterocolitis
bowel perforation 157
ileostomy after 157
twin-to-twin tranfusion causing 19
Neomycin, for conjunctivitis 22
Neonatal lupus syndrome 37
Neonatal tumours
adrenal 165
Langerhans cell histiocytosis 168–9
neuroblastoma and skin nodules 166
pharyngel teratoma 171
renal tumour 167
sacro-coccygeal teratoma 172
Neuroblastoma
radiograph showing 165
skin nodules associated 166
Neurofibromatosis type 1, 82
Neurology
anencephaly 76
arachnoid cyst 84
bilateral open-lipped schizencephaly 86
cerebral function monitor 83
congenital aqueduct stenosis 78
corpus collosum agenesis 85
encephalocoele 78
hydrocephalus 77
hypotonia 81
hypoxic ischaemic damage to basal ganglia 84
microcephaly 75
multiple intraventricular haemorrhages 85
neurofibromatosis 82
spina bifida 79
occulta 80
thoracic meningomyelocoele 80
Niemann–Pick disease 54
Nose
dermoid cyst 62
haemangioma 27

O

Oesophageal atresia 95, 124
Oils 16
Oligohydramnios 127
Omphalocoele 101
Optic glioma 82
Osteogenesis imperfecta 130–1

Oxygen probe monitor, ischaemia after 178–9

P

Paronychia, staphylococcal skin sepsis 15
Pericardial effusion 87
Perineum
  acrodermatitis enteropathica 42
  Candida 16
Peritoneal calcification 107
Pharyngeal teratoma 171
Phosphate supplements 132
Phototherapy, for jaundice 21
Pierre Robin sequence 68
  feeding, Haberman teat 69–70
  tracheostomy 70
Plagiocephaly, occipital 50–1
Pneumatosis intestinalis 157
Pneumonia
  congenital 92–3
  and conjunctivitis 22
  pneumocystis 35
Pneumothorax 154–5
Polycythaemia 19, 20
  infant of diabetes mother 150
Polydactyly 123
  and brachycephaly 53
Port wine stain 29
Potter syndrome 145
Preterm babies
  bronchopulmonary dysplasia 153
  dehydration 158
  flow driver 164
  hand, scarring of previous 180
  intracranial bleeds 159–64
  necrotizing enterocolitis 157
  pneumothorax 154
  pulmonary interstitial emphysema 152
  respiratory distress syndrome 151, 154
Proptosis 58
Pseudoachrondroplasia 122
Ptosis 56
Pulmonary interstitial emphysema 152
Pulmonary venous drainage obstruction, total anomalous 96
Purpura
  congenital CMV, 43
  Langerhans cell histiocytosis 169

R

Rectal agenesis 108–9
Red reflex 57
Renal tumour, congenital 167
Respiratory distress syndrome
  bronchopulmonary dysplasia after 153
  ground-glass appearance 151
  pneumothorax after 154
Rhesus disease, hydrops foetalis 90
Rickets, and hypotonia 81
Robinow (fetal face) syndrome 145
Rubella, congenital
  cataract due to 57
  microcephaly due to 75
Russell–Silver dwarfism
  body appearance 143
  facies 143

S

Sacral agenesis
  infant of diabetes mother 150
  rocker bottom feet and 122
Sacral area, blue spots 30–1
Sacro-coccygeal teratoma 172
Sandal gap 141
Scalp
  cradle cap 16
  oils for 12, 16
  strawberry naevus 25
Scaphocephaly 47
Schizencephaly, bilateral open-lipped 86
Seborrhoeic dermatitis 12–13
  with *Candida* 13
  and cradle cap 16
Sepsis
  congenital gram-negative 43
  group beta streptococcal 93
  jaundice due to 21
Shoulder dystocia 6
Shoulder presentation 5, 6
Skeletal disorders
  amniotic bands 118–20
  arthrogryposis 127
  camptomelic dysplasia 126
  club feet 117
  club hand 124
  congenital tail 136
  metatarsus adductus varus 121
  osteogenesis imperfecta 131
  polydactyly 124
  rickets 132
  rocker bottom feet 122
  skeletal dysplasia 122–3
  split hand and foot syndrome 128–9
  Sprengel's deformity 134
  syndactyly 125
  talipes calcaneovalgus 120
  tumoral calcinosis 133
Skeletal dysplasia 122–3
Skin
acrodermatitis enteropathica 42
annular erythema 35
  blue spots 30–1
  collodion baby 32
  congenital melanocytic naevus 24
    giant 23
  congenital varicella 44–5
  cradle cap 16
  cytomegalovirus 43
  dermoid cyst 62
  disseminated haemangiomatosis 34
  eczema herpeticum 40
  epidermal naevus 33
  epidermolysis bullosa 36
  erythema toxicum 10–11
  extensive haemangioma 26–7
  gram-negative sepsis 43
  incontinentia pigmenti 33
  Langerhans cell histiocytosis-related rash 168–9
  lupus syndrome 37
  milia 9
  milk allergy 40
  neonatal herpes 46
  neuroblastoma-associated nodules 166
  port wine stain 28–9
  pre-auricular tags 64
  seborrhoeic dermatitis 12–13
  staphylococcal sepsis 14–15
  strawberry naevi 24–5
  toxic epidermal necrolysis 37
  water loss 158
Skull
  brachycephaly 53
  fracture and cephalohaematoma 1
  plagiocephaly 50–1
  trigonocephaly 52
  wormian bones 131
Spina bifida 79
  and club foot 117
  occulta 80
Spinal abnormalities, epidermal naevus 33
Spinal cord tumours 82
Split hand and foot syndrome 129
Spondyloepiphyseal dysplasia 122
Sprengel's deformity 134
Staphylococcal skin sepsis 11, 14–15
Sternomastoid tumour 72
Steroids
  with antifungals, for Candida 13, 16
  for seborrheic dermatitis 12
  for infantile eczema 39

Stools
  of breast-fed babies 115
  green 115
  and meconium 115
  necrotizing enterocolitis 157
  and normal bowel-opening 115
  pale, of conjugated jaundice 105
Sturge-Weber syndrome 29
  and glaucoma 58
Subglottal stenosis, endotracheal intubation causing 70
Syndactyly 125
  and brachycephaly 53
Systemic lupus erythematosus 35

T

Tail, congenital 136
Talipes calcaneovalgus, bilateral 120
Talipes equinovarus, bilateral 117
TAR syndrome 124
Tay-Sachs disease 54
Teeth, neonatal 20
Thromboctyopaenia
  and CMV, 43
  and absence of radius (TAR syndrome) 124
  and extensive haemangiomas in Kasabach–Merritt syndrome 27
  and large naevi 27
  lupus syndrome causing 37
  in neonatal herpes 46
  twin-to-twin tranfusion causing 19
  in Wiskott–Aldrich syndrome 146
Thyroxine therapy 147
Tibial artery catheter, gangrene after 174
Tongue
  glossoptosis 73
  macroglossia 73
Total parenteral nutrition burns 176
Toxic epidermal necrolysis 37
Toxoplasmosis, congenital 60
Tracheo-oesophageal atresia, in VATER complex 124
Tracheo-oesophageal fistula 95
Tracheostomy 70
Transient tachypnoea of the newborn 96
Treacher Collins syndrome 65
  absent ear 63
  facies 65
Trigonocephaly 52
Trisomy 13
  anophthalmos and 55
  and coloboma 57
Trisomy 18 *see* Edward syndrome
Tumoral calcinosis 133
Turner syndrome 144
  rocker bottom feet and 122
  skeletal dysplasia 122
Twins
  acute fetofetal transfusion 20
  post-haemorrhagic hydrocephalus 77
  Siamese 137
  transfusion syndrome 19
Tyrosinaemia 105

U

Umbilical granuloma 101
  differential diagnosis 99
  silver nitrate burn 180
Umbilical hernia 100–1
Upper limb, haemangioma 27
Uterus, thickened 149

V

Varicella, congenital 45
VATER complex 124
Ventouse extraction
  cephalohaematoma 1
  misshapen head 2
  skin marks 2
Vitello-intestinal duct, persistence 99
Vomiting, bile-stained
  anal stenosis with obstruction 108
  duodenal atresia 98
  duodenal web and malrotation 97
Vulval oedema 177

W

Werdnig–Hoffman 81
Wilm's tumour 59, 142
Wiskott–Aldrich syndrome 146
Wormian bones 131

Z

Zinc deficiency 42